friday's footprint

Friday's Footprint

HOW SOCIETY SHAPES THE HUMAN MIND

Leslie Brothers

New York   Oxford
Oxford University Press
1997

Oxford University Press

Oxford New York
Athens Auckland Bangkok Bogotá Bombay
Buenos Aires Calcutta Cape Town Dar es Salaam
Delhi Florence Hong Kong Istanbul Karachi
Kuala Lumpur Madras Madrid Melbourne
Mexico City Nairobi Paris Singapore
Taipei Tokyo Toronto

and associated companies in
Berlin Ibadan

Copyright © 1997 by Oxford University Press, Inc.

Published by Oxford University Press, Inc.
198 Madison Avenue, New York, New York 10016

Oxford is a registered trademark of Oxford University Press, Inc.

Library of Congress Cataloging-in-Publication Data
Brothers, Leslie.
Friday's footprint: how society shapes the human mind / Leslie Brothers
p.   cm.
Includes bibliographical references and index.
ISBN 0–19–510103–0
1. Cognition—Social aspects. 2. Cognition and culture. 3. Human
information processing—Social aspects. I. Title.
BF311.B75 1997
153—dc21   97-13482

1 3 5 7 9 8 6 4 2

Printed in the United States of America
on acid-free paper

This book is dedicated to Bruce

. . . he spoke some words to me; and though I could not understand them, yet I thought they were pleasant to hear; for they were the first sound of a man's voice that I had heard, my own excepted, for above twenty-five years. . . . In a little time I began to speak to him. . . ; and, first, I made him know his name should be Friday, which was the day I saved his life.

—Daniel Defoe, *Robinson Crusoe*

Contents

Preface

How does brain activity give rise to human experience? How does it allow us to have selves, to speak poetically or persuasively, and to treat others as persons rather than things? Many solutions to this problem have been put forward; woven into them is an assumption that appears again and again, expressed in a variety of ways. It holds that although brain activity is the engine of human behavior, the *forms* that human experience takes are designed by culture. Like the intricate designs set in wax by a royal seal, thought arises from biological matter through the impress of culture. Conceived in this way, there is an unexplained gulf between biology and culture, a gulf that—for scientists, at least—attracts efforts to bridge the two and so unify the world under the aegis of the natural sciences. This book is such an attempt.

The classic fictional story *Robinson Crusoe* describes how a shipwrecked sailor survived alone on a desert island. He prayed, kept a diary, and industriously made tools, clothing, and shelter for himself. This image of the isolated individual embodies a metaphor for the human mind; it is the metaphor that has determined the practices of contemporary neuroscience—until now. To bridge the worlds of brain and mind, we will replace this isolated mind metaphor with a view that is thoroughly social.

What is more, we will put old observations in a new perspective. The following parallel from the history of biology illustrates how a shift in perspective leads to understanding. In the seventeenth and eighteenth centuries, biologists were at a loss as to how to explain the development of complex organisms from apparently simple eggs and sperm. The two opposing camps in that controversy consisted of the preformationists on the one hand, who believed a tiny adult must somehow reside within the egg or sperm (a conjecture whose truth never could be demonstrated); and the vitalists on the other, who held that gradual differentiation of complex structure was attributable to some mystical, vital force. In the latter half of the nineteenth century, chemical stains and microscopes revealed to biologists' curious eyes a heavily stained material in cell nuclei, material that was named *chromatin*. Little by little, as more analytic methods became available, chromatin was induced to give up its secrets. Ultimately, the deoxyribonucleic acid (DNA) it contained was described and understood. And once DNA's structure, and then its function, were unravelled, the physical basis of the previously mysterious processes of inheritance and differentiation could be explained. To achieve this outcome, techniques for seeing chromatin had to be developed, and the importance of chromatin in inheritance had to be grasped. Today, we know that eggs and sperm have *blueprints* for structure: although lacking organs themselves, they carry instructions, in the form of DNA, for the subsequent differentiation of the embryo's many organs. Now we know how the instructions are read, transcribed, and turned into the amazing variety of proteins that make up differentiated organisms. Because we understand these mechanisms, we no longer have use for theoretical debates regarding tiny, invisible entities or mystical forces. The problem has been reconceptualized.

Similarly, to bridge the gap between minds and brains, we must grasp the significance of observations already available to us. We take the first step by acknowledging that the network of meanings we call culture arises from the *joint* activities of human brains. This network forms the living content of the mind, so that the mind is communal in its very nature: It cannot be derived from any single brain in isolation. By developing several strands of evidence from several disciplines, we then begin to see how brains work jointly to make culture. One strand addresses the human brain's inborn mechanism for generating and perceiving "person," a construct that assigns individuals subjectivity. Another concerns the particularities of persons, selves, and the social order, and how these are continually mediated and defined in that deceptively humble behavior, conversation—behavior for which our brains have evolved by elaborating on neural mechanisms for more ancient forms of communication. We will close the circle by noting how social systems of belief, conveyed through public acts and narratives, are taken up and reproduced in individual behavior. Just as chromatin proved to hold the key to the mystery of inheritance, human conversation holds the key to the mind. The characteristics of conversation, its role in human society, and its roots in brain function are the subject of this work.

The book is organized as follows. Chapter 1 introduces the concept of person and illustrates how it can be altered or lost in cases of brain disorder. An important aspect of the concept of person is the idea of "mental life." In chapter 2, researchers' findings on how we attribute mental lives to others are reviewed. Then, chapter 3 introduces the remarkable findings of neurophysiologists that first hinted at a primate specialization for social communication. These discoveries, together with data derived from observing monkeys in captivity and in the wild, form the unfolding story of "the social brain." Having begun to understand how the brain makes sense of the actions of others, we are prepared for chapter 4's look at fascinating evidence from patients undergoing electrical brain stimulation. Chapter 5 shifts the focus to the scientific community, examining the tension between the new, social framework for brain research and the old, isolated mind metaphor.

Conversation is our species' vehicle for creating the concepts of person and society. Thus, chapter 6 turns to conversation, drawing on the work of conversation researchers to demonstrate the highly structured nature of human conversation. Reviewing evidence from studies that compare the anatomy of several species, we see that the primate brain evolved to send and receive facial gestures, and now deploys these as an essential part of discourse. In both ancient and modern forms of communication, the interchange of expressions is a jointly created performance whose nature is essentially public. Performances, together with narratives, are used by communities to establish consensual realities. In chapter 7 we learn more of the mechanisms of "common sense," including how the commonsense notion of self arises.

But common sense can fool us. In chapter 8 I show that the commonsense concept of emotion belongs to the realm of everyday thought, but surprisingly, this does not hold up as a useful category in neuroscience. Nevertheless, our experiences are determined by the everyday concepts to which we subscribe through participating in collective narratives and performances. This key tenet is illustrated in chapter 9. There I show how psychoanalysis, a variant of everyday culture that uses a specialized kind of conversation, can create new experiences of self.

Chapter 10 summarizes some of the implications of the book's arguments. Although in our everyday language we often refer to aspects of "mind," nothing in that language can be mapped directly onto the brain. When the language of natural science turns to the human brain's evolved capacity for social interaction, however, we open up an entirely new perspective. In social interactions, human beings invent and develop vocabularies of motivation and experience. When neuroscience takes up these interactions, the natural sciences, which are concerned with causes, and the human sciences, which are concerned with reasons, are united within a single framework.

With the closing chapter, we are ready to view Robinson Crusoe in a new light. He was never isolated, for he came to his desert island carrying with him all the conversations and narratives of his society. His eventual discovery of the traces of another human being is akin to the discovery of socially responsive neurons in the brains of primates. This book reinterprets both as "discoveries" in the truest sense, because they were there all the time—they reveal the essentially social nature of mind.

September 1996   L. B.
Los Angeles, California

Acknowledgments

I am very grateful to a number of individuals who have contributed in important ways to the writing of this book. Elinor Ochs introduced me to ethnomethodology and conversation analysis. An anonymous reviewer directed me to Strawson's essay. Alan Bond, Simon Baron-Cohen, Jochen Braun, Arthur Kling, and Robert Perinbanayagam provided valuable comments on the manuscript. I received helpful comments on an early draft of the chapter on psychoanalysis from Marcia Cavell, Victoria Hamilton, George Pigman, and Robert Stolorow, and on a later draft from Ulrich Streeck.

Joan Bossert, my editor, has provided excellent guidance. Many others, working in various organizations, have been helpful as well. The UCLA Library has been an outstanding resource. The Veterans Administration Hospital at Sepulveda, through its Psychiatry Division, has supported my efforts throughout this project. The Institute of Contemporary Psychoanalysis has provided an atmosphere of intellectual openness that has been invaluable.

I am fortunate in having a friend who is both an advocate and an unflinching critic: Jochen Braun (Achim) has been both, to the great benefit of my writing.

I am indebted beyond expression to Arthur Kling, for years of generous, patient support.

My husband, Alan Bond, encouraged me to write this book in the first place. Our many discussions have found places within it. They have made it much better than it would otherwise have been.

Although those I have named deserve credit for any strengths the work may have, they are not responsible for its flaws, limitations, and errors.

Finally, I thank Sarah and Robin for their love and forbearance.

friday's footprint

1

A Failure to Connect

Introducing "Person"

Let me begin with three accounts that have a common theme.

In one, a woman was brought to an emergency room by her relatives. She denied having any illness, and went on to tell the doctor that there was a man living in her house who looked just like her husband—but she knew he was not in actuality her husband.

For the second account, I quote a pair of neurologists writing in 1989:

A 77-year-old woman (S.M.) began to develop visual disturbances and forgetfulness. She also developed the belief that there was another S.M. who was identical to herself in appearance, age, background, education, etc. This other S.M. was always seen in a mirror. If the patient's son or the examiner appeared behind the patient in the mirror the patient would correctly label their mirror reflection. Thus, the phenomenon was only evident for her own image. The misidentification was most likely to occur when the patient looked at the mirror in her own bedroom, but could occur in the examiner's office as well as in mirrors in other locations. When it was pointed out to the patient that this was indeed her own mirror image, the patient would say to her son, "Oh sure, that's what you think."[1]

For the third account, I quote a pediatrician who wrote the following about certain children seen in his practice:

The children's relation to people is altogether different. Every one of the children upon entering the office immediately went after blocks, toys, or other objects without paying the least attention to the persons present. It would be wrong to say that they were not aware of the presence of persons. But the people, as long as they left the child alone, figured in about the same manner as did the desk, the bookshelf, or the filing cabinet.[2]

What these fascinating cases have in common are the patients' inability to attach appropriate mental lives to the bodies around them. In the first example, the body of the husband was believed not to have the mind of the husband. In the second example, the body seen in the mirror was perceived not as a mere reflection, but as a person with a mind. In the third example, the children behaved as if other individuals were only bodies, without mental lives at all. All these patients have very unusual ways of connecting minds and bodies. As we explore the worlds of such individuals in this chapter, it will begin to become apparent how it is that we construct our usual, everyday perceptions of "persons."

What do we mean by "person"? First, we mean a being with a mental life, an "owner" of conscious subjective experience. The mental life of the individual we each call "I"—ourselves—seems one of the most simple and unarguable facts of existence. Yet philosophers such as Alfred Ayer and Peter Strawson have argued at length about the *logic* of bodies "having" subjective experience.[3] One of Strawson's key ideas was that the person concept—the union of a mental life with a body— is logically "primitive," by which he meant that the concept of a mental life derives from the concept of person, not the other way around. My account of how our brains work supports his idea. In my account, "person" is a higher level perception of bodies, a perception that endows them with mental life. We endow bodies with mental life in the same way we endow the sights or sounds of words with meaning, which is what gives them their semantic, as opposed to their phonetic, dimension. Because of the way our brains work, our perception of "person" is automatic. It is an obligatory part of our experience of others—and ourselves.

But there is another dimension to the concept "person"—a person always belongs in a network of persons, a network that has been termed the "social order."[4] The social order is intrinsically moral, for it is made up of shoulds and oughts, triumph and shame, villains and heroes. Personal behavior in this moral-social order is interpreted in terms of reasons and shifting status. How this dimension of the person concept is created and negotiated in everyday interaction is the subject of chapter 6.

Returning to the relation between our perception of bodies and our perception of persons, let's elaborate on the idea that perceiving "person" is obligatory. I will again resort to language as an analogy. When I hear a word in a language I know, it is not possible for me to hear *just* the sounds. I am compelled to experience the meaning of the word, its semantic aspect. In the same way that words are made of lower level features, such as sounds or symbols, persons are made of features like body appearance, body movement, voice, and face. When we see or hear one of these features, we are compelled to experience it as indicative of the presence of a person who has both subjectivity and a location in the social order—whether we happen to know the person's identity or not.[5]

Some have taken the position that the person concept is entirely an artifact of culture. Strawson, for example, pointed out that an intrinsic part of the person concept is the idea of a "self" that somehow owns subjective experience. He pointed out how strange this is, as it is an ownership that cannot be transferred, violating the very sense of the concept of ownership. He concluded therefore that the idea of person must derive from a linguistic illusion. In other words, he argued, we have it because we are members of a language community. Communities elaborate their own informal, nonscientific theories of behavior, sometimes referred to as "folk psychology." The psychologist Jerome Bruner wrote, "Personhood is itself a constituent concept of our folk psychology."[6]

But I am not convinced that the person concept is an arbitrary result of cultural learning. Culture certainly has an impact on its content, and its impact will occupy us at length later on. The point here, though, is that human beings are biologically prepared to subscribe to the concept of person just as we are biologically prepared to learn a language. There is a neural basis for representations of persons, for cases such as those we have seen result from disturbed brain function or abnormalities of brain development.

Liberace and the Pope

Certain aphasic patients—individuals whose language has been disrupted by brain injury—may correctly hear the sounds of words although they are unable to perceive their meanings. The perception of persons can also be disrupted by brain injury in ways that parallel this language deficit of aphasia: These disorders, which are documented mainly in psychiatric reports, are called "misidentification syndromes."

Patients suffering from misidentification syndromes may lose the ability to experience another as a being with a mental life, although the perception of the person's body remains intact. For example, the sufferer may perceive a "zombie" or, in a milder form, a strange person inhabiting a familiar body. This kind of disorder occurs in individuals suffering from Capgras syndrome, an uncommon but by no means rare phenomenon that may be seen in psychiatric patients, or in medical patients with localized brain dysfunction. Such a patient might complain, as in the example at the beginning of the chapter, "There is a man living in my house who looks just like my husband, but I know he is not my husband." The experience of Capgras syndrome is created for moviegoers in the film *Invasion of the Body Snatchers*. In such patients, lower level descriptions (about the body or its identity) remain intact, but the semantic level (the person) is lost.

Individuals suffering from the poorly understood spectrum of disorders called schizophrenia frequently experience the deterioration of semantic-level representations, sometimes for *both* language and the concept of person. In the sphere of language, this results in using words for their sounds rather than for their meanings. For example, a hospitalized schizophrenic patient approached me and said, "Dr. Brothers, are you my brother?" This use of language has been called "klang association" and has been observed by generations of psychiatrists.

The following case illustrates an analogous breakdown in the semantic category of person, in which the patient resorts to lower level representation—namely, descriptions of bodily appearance. It involves a patient I interviewed, the woman who was brought to the emergency room by her relatives because she was convinced that a look-alike imposter had been substituted for her real husband. When I questioned her, she told me not only about the substitution, but also her theory as to why it was taking place. She speculated that there was a mysterious worldwide plot afoot, involving a collaboration between Liberace (a popular pianist often seen on television in the 1950s and 1960s, notable for his flashy attire) and the Pope. To a listener, such a conjunction seems at first ludicrous, for in our taken-for-granted social order, there could hardly be two persons who have less to do with one another. But when one turns to the level of the bodily representation and focuses on their ornate, jewel-encrusted garments, a similarity becomes oddly apparent. Like patients using "klang" associations between words, the woman did not have access to the semantics of person and social order. She made connections based on physical characteristics instead.

Problems in person cognition may spill over to invade the representation of the body as well, just as some kinds of aphasia involve not only semantics, but also word forms. The words that are produced in what is called Wernicke's aphasia, for example, are either nonsubstantive, incorrect approximations of appropriate words, or pure nonsense. Wernicke's aphasia involves both word features (sounds) and their semantic counterparts (meaning). Similarly, some misidentification syndromes involve both body representations and their semantic counterparts:

persons. To illustrate this observation, let's turn to another account, this one of a patient suffering from a misidentification syndrome.

> A 37-year-old psychiatric patient, Mr. F., had been jailed for getting in a fight. While in jail he was visited by his sister. Mr. F. accepted her as his sister but believed her face was different than his sister's—it was "unrecognizable" and "of a different age."
>
> The patient believed that copies of his mind had been placed in the bodies of different people who had been previously unknown to him. He perceived some other visitors to the jail as having undergone both physical and psychological transformations, for example, they had distorted bodies, enlarged heads, and alien minds.[7]

Is it significant that the people in these cases display derangements in representations of both body and person? We will return to this intriguing question later in this chapter.

The syndromes described here encompass various colorful disorders sometimes named for the neurologists who first recognized them. We have just seen that a syndrome may involve primarily the perception of person, or a mixture of body and person. Another way of categorizing the syndromes is according to whether they involve others, the self, or both.[8]

In Capgras syndrome, the individual suffers from the delusion that a person has been somehow transformed (not himself), while his physical body remains constant: "This woman looks just like my mother, but she is not: my mother has been replaced by an imposter." In Frégoli syndrome, the delusion is that another's psychological identity is preserved, whereas the physical identity is altered: "My teacher appeared yesterday as my boss; last night as my brother; now he is masquerading as my doctor." The syndrome of intermetamorphosis is characterized by delusions regarding both the physical body and a person's identity: "My sister is a space creature; half of her body is transparent."

Delusions of the self also occur. In the syndrome of subjective doubles, the patient believes that others, who are psychologically different, take on his or her own physical characteristics: "I have been seeing look-alikes of myself." In the syndrome of reverse subjective doubles, the individual believes that he or she is being transformed into someone else's psychological identity: "An imposter is taking over my body." And in the syndrome of reverse intermetamorphosis, the patient believes he or she is changing both psychologically and physically: "I have changed into a woman—a prostitute," states a male patient. "I am having labor pains and am about to deliver a baby." Patients may even believe that parts of their body are dead, or not real, as in Cotard syndrome.

In all of these syndromes, the patients' explanations for their perceptions are also delusional. They invoke plots, aliens, demonic possession, and incredible details to explain the phenomena they are experiencing. The best way to understand the core problem is to disregard the rationalizations and consider the misperceptions along two axes: body/person and self/other.

Two interesting features of these syndromes deserve mention. One is that they frequently occur in combination, that is, an individual suffering from Capgras syndrome may also complain of several other misidentification symptoms, as in the previous case of Mr. F. This alerts us to the probability that all these syndromes have a common neural basis, whether they concern the physical or psychological identity, and whether they concern the self or others. It corroborates the assertion that psychological entities (persons) are linked preferentially to bodies under normal conditions, just as the meanings of words are linked to their sounds, so that a single disruption in neural processes affects both representations. Wernicke's aphasia illustrates this principle in the domain of language. The fact that both self and other can be involved also corroborates Strawson's purely theoretical point that the notion of person irreducibly applies both to others and to self, that is, it is essential to the character of person predicates that they have both first- and third-person ascriptive uses.

The second point worth noting about these phenomena is that they are associated with brain dysfunction. (See Figure 1.1 for a depiction of brain structures mentioned in this section.) Patients with right parietal lobe lesions may deny that the left half of their body is impaired, even in the presence of obvious paralysis, or they may deny that the affected body parts are their own. Delusions affecting psychological aspects of the self may occur in the presence of temporal lobe lesions. For example, a patient with a calcification in the left temporal lobe complained of a "feeling of being another person." Another patient with a cavernous angioma (malformation of the blood vessels) of the right temporal lobe said, "I felt as if another person was going to take possession of my brain; as if I were on the TV."[9]

Most brain lesions that give rise to these phenomena are more diffuse than the ones just mentioned, however. A patient with a typical constellation of psychotic symptoms (including, for example, auditory hallucinations and loose associations) developed the conviction that a taxi driver, a salesman, a pedestrian, and a priest were all in fact Mr. B., her theology instructor, whom she believed was in love with her. She also had episodes in which her body became "light as a feather." After some psychological tests, it became apparent that the woman

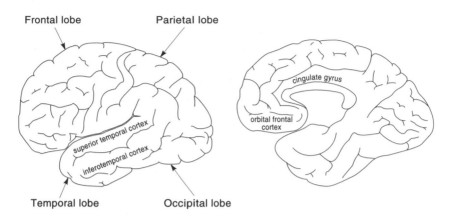

Figure 1.1   The human brain in lateral view, as if the head were in profile with the nose pointing left. (*left*) A lateral view—that is, looking from the outside at one of the brain's hemispheres. Major lobes of the brain are indicated, together with some subregions of the temporal lobe's cortex. (*right*) A medial view—that is, a view of one hemisphere from the inside.

had diffuse brain dysfunction, which was corroborated by the finding of epileptic-like activity in both temporal lobes. Such findings are typical for these disorders. For example, a brain scan of the 77-year-old woman who misidentified her mirror reflection showed evidence of mild generalized decrease in brain volume, with right temporal and parietal loss in particular. An electroencephalogram (an EEG, used to measure brain waves) showed that this woman had cerebral dysfunction of both left and right hemispheres, with accentuation on the right.

Localized or diffuse, it is generally accepted that brain dysfunction is the cause of misidentification syndromes. In one series of 15 cases of intermetamorphosis syndrome, 9 had known histories of head injury, substance abuse, or epilepsy. For example, Mr. F., whose case was described above, had had a seizure disorder since age 14. A man who had the conviction that he had been transformed into a woman and was about to deliver a baby had developed his symptoms after suffering a head injury. A patient with an encapsulated parasitic lesion in the left temporal lobe developed Capgras syndrome at the onset of his treatment. But despite attempts to localize brain areas that result in misidentification, no simple picture has emerged. This suggests that the representation of the body and especially of the person—one's own mental life or someone else's—is encoded in widespread regions of the brain. These representations may become altered either in the case of widespread dysfunction, or when lesions in linking areas, such as regions of the temporal lobes, are combined with dysfunction elsewhere, especially in the right hemisphere, and perhaps in the parietal lobe in particular.[10]

The fact that representations of both body and person are linked suggests that a brain system that originally evolved for registering social features of a physical kind underwent a further elaboration—perhaps only a slight one—to yield representations of mental life. We know of other organ systems in which slight modifications of existing structures gave rise to new capacities as a result of nature's persistent tinkering. The vision scientist Vilayanur Ramachandran observed,

> Nature is inherently opportunistic and will often adopt some very curious—even bizarre—solutions to its problems, especially when it has to make use of pre-existing hardware. To appreciate this point, consider the three tiny bones in our middle ear which are used to amplify sounds. In the reptilian antecedents of mammals these same three bones constitute part of the hinge mechanism of the lower jaw, used for chewing food. Thus what was originally part of the reptilian lower jaw used for mastication, has now been incorporated into the mammalian middle ear to be used in hearing![11]

Our prehuman ancestors possessed neural systems that had been gradually adapted for detecting and responding to the sights and sounds of their fellow primates (systems we shall learn more about in later chapters). I suggest that, just as reptilian jaw bones migrated gradually to give rise to an organ that could register sounds, socially dedicated neural systems were progressively organized during our evolution to give rise to a neural organ that could generate the experience of "mind."

What would happen if such an organ were damaged? We are so accustomed to attaching minds to bodies that it is hard for us to imagine what it is like not to construct the experience of mind. That is one reason why the clinical reports above are so valuable. The minds that the patients would normally have constructed to accompany their own or others' bodies became disconnected or distorted. As a result, their experiences of "person" were devastatingly altered. Imagining the strangeness of these experiences is a way to bring our normal, everyday construction of mind into focus.

These reports are informative in another way. I am suggesting that our ancestors began with a brain system specialized for perceiving and responding to bodies and their gestures, and that a slight modification of this system enabled us to generate the percepts of person and mind.

If my idea is correct, then disordered activity in these circuits would be expected to affect the perception of both bodily features and mental lives—and we have seen that this is the case. These reports, then, provide us with important clues as to the nature of the brain system that constructs our experience of mind.

Missing Persons

We have just considered the consequences of damage to brain systems that control our ability to construct a "mind." Another way that these systems can go awry is for the capacity to be missing from birth as a result of an inborn brain abnormality. Because our brain capacities and structures are elaborated sequentially during development, the manifestations of an innate disorder are usually different from those of an acquired disorder. We now turn to an innate disorder—autism.

Early infantile autism was first described by Leo Kanner, a pediatrician, in 1944. The children he described had unusual social interactions, in that they seemed indifferent to other people, or would approach others only in order to have physical needs met. He wrote the description quoted at the beginning of this chapter in order to convey that his young patients related to others very much as though they were pieces of furniture rather than persons.

Kanner's patients had, in addition, odd ways of communicating. Although their language was grammatically correct, it was often literal and idiosyncratic, or it might consist simply of repetitions of the words and phrases they heard. Sometimes pronouns were used inappropriately, for example, by a child's referring to himself as "he" rather than "I." Unlike other children, autistic children did not play by elaborating pretend scenarios, or if they were able to play, their use of imagination would be quite limited and wouldn't include people. They often engaged in repetitive acts: they might rock, or tap themselves continuously, and they might spin or manipulate objects in a monotonous way. Their interests tended to be narrow, and often nonsocial; for example, timetables or arithmetic would be engrossing for these children. A need for strict routines was occasionally seen, with any changes in routine causing temper tantrums. Finally, it was sometimes the case that such children might have a single, unusual skill, such as drawing, calculating, or music, developed to a level well beyond their mental age, although they remained very impaired in other skills.

This description has been upheld to the present day as constituting a cluster of symptoms, some or all of which may be present, in varying degrees of severity, in certain children. Like Kanner, contemporary researchers emphasize the social deficits of autism, holding these to be essential for diagnosing the syndrome. The prevalence of the full syndrome of impairments as described by Kanner is estimated to be about 2 to 4 children in 10,000; if we look at the prevalence of just the core syndrome alone—the social impairments—the prevalence climbs to about 15 to 20 children in 10,000.[12]

The causes of autism may vary. It has been associated with genetic factors, as well as with a variety of intrauterine events, such as infections. A derangement of the normal development and migration of neurons during the first 6 months may be the underlying mechanism for the brain abnormalities that have been observed in autism, although other causes have been proposed as well. Although various events may result in brain abnormalities during gestation, not all children with brain damage are autistic. Therefore, it is thought that the syndrome will only arise if particular brain areas or functions involved in *social* abilities are affected. (We look in more detail at the neuropathological findings in autism in chapter 4.)

To understand autism, we need to understand some general features of brain function. All our human senses are at the disposal of forces with powerful interests, much like newspapers in a country ruled by a dictator. If you read those newspapers, it is true that you are getting an account of the world, a series of reports. We like to think of the brain as an unbiased, neutral reporter. But the fact is the reports from our senses are produced in collaboration with other brain regions, regions trained over evolutionary time to act as editors in the service of powerful special interests—social ones. As a primate, having access to mates or rearing one's offspring successfully requires biased control over the cortical media. One's brain must select and report on *social* events— the more quickly and accurately, the better.

How does the brain select and report on social events normally? From the beginning, human infants attend to social stimuli, suggesting that inborn brain mechanisms direct them toward the sights and sounds of other human beings. As a result of this predilection, they receive a steady stream of social information, and neural assemblies representing social objects flourish. Several experiments reveal that social objects are interesting to infants.

From birth, human infants pay preferential attention to visual stimuli that look like human faces (see Figure 1.2). Very young newborns can imitate facial expressions, indicating that their visual systems are able to perceive such elements as raised or furrowed eyebrows and open mouths. By a slightly older age, infants associate voices with faces: 1- to 2-month-old infants are distressed by the spatial separation

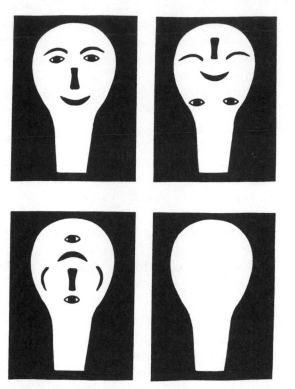

Figure 1.2   Stimuli that were shown to a group of forty newborn infants, median age 9 minutes. The infants were much more likely to turn their heads and eyes so as to follow the face-like stimulus, than they were to follow the scrambled or blank stimuli. (From "Visual following and pattern discrimination of face-like stimuli by newborn infants" by C. Goren, M. Sarty, and P. Wu [1975]. Pediatrics, 56, p. 545. Reproduced by permission of *Pediatrics*. Copyright © 1975 by *Pediatrics*.)

of face and voice, indicating that they "know," either from experience or innately, that voices are supposed to issue from faces. Interestingly, though, when a face "talks," it is not the mouth that attracts an infant's attention. In one study, 7- to 11-week-old infants looking at adult faces showed a tendency to shift their gaze to the region of the eyes when the face was talking, compared to when it was silent. Although the tendency was only slight, the finding is significant because it is the opposite of what one might have expected: one might have expected that the infants' attention would be attracted primarily by movement, and therefore by the mouth, rather than the eye region. The observation therefore suggests that an infant's attention is drawn to the *expressive* movements in the region around the eyes when speech is underway.

"Motherese," the exaggeratedly expressive facial and vocal signals that human adults in all cultures instinctively direct toward babies, may be the adult's adaptation to the infant's preference for expressiveness in face and voice.[13]

Because of our innate attraction to the sights and sounds of faces, we probably have a considerable amount of neural circuitry devoted to faces by the end of our first year of life. And all this brain machinery makes us remarkably expert when it comes to faces. For example, we can identify many different faces, even though as a class faces are all quite similar visually. In addition, we readily notice subtle changes in facial expression, as was demonstrated in an experiment in which research subjects were able to detect very tiny differences between similar computerized line drawings depicting facial expressions. We are also extremely acute when it comes to detecting another's gaze direction. Finally, we automatically use information from the sight of mouth movements to understand speech, even without formal instruction in lipreading.[14]

How does language learning relate to the perception of facial and vocal expression? Although they appear to develop together in infancy, by the time adulthood is reached, neural ensembles for perceiving and producing language become somewhat separate from those specialized for perceiving and producing expressions. Usually, the left hemisphere is specialized for linguistic functions, and the right for emotionally expressive ones. This is true regardless of whether the sensory modality in which emotional or linguistic stimuli are presented is visual or auditory. In the visual case, for example, lipreading appears to depend more on left-sided mechanisms, as does the integration of seen and heard speech, whereas interpretation of emotional facial gestures depends more on right-sided mechanisms. In the auditory case, understanding and producing emotional intonation of speech appears to depend more on the right hemisphere, whereas linguistic understanding and production depend on the left. Although language-related left-hemisphere sites are activated earlier and more strongly than corresponding right-hemisphere sites by tasks in which subjects view and then name pictures of everyday objects, it is also apparent that the right hemisphere is quite active during this task. This observation warns us not to adopt an extreme view of the hemispheres as functionally separate. In general, however, the right hemisphere seems to have an advantage for registering the expressive aspects of human communication.[15]

The brain's representations of facial and vocal expressiveness form the developmental core of the representation we call "person." The implications of research on the infant's earliest exposure to speech suggest that these sounds engage brain mechanisms that register *expressions*—both vocal and facial—preferentially. We saw earlier that misidentification syndromes are more often associated with right-hemisphere damage. If expression and a concept of person are indeed linked as right-hemisphere representations, then the infant's earliest perceptions of linguistic utterances—expressive sounds—are anchored in representations of a person. In other words, the child does not attach utterances to persons because of logical, abstract necessity. Instead, utterances are intrinsically attached to persons because language perception shares the same neural ensembles that encode expressive faces and voices. Later, as the two hemispheres specialize in linguistic and expressive signaling, respectively, both systems are engaged simultaneously.

Understanding utterances, and attributing them to a person as their source, are fundamentally intertwined. It is the *intentions of speakers* that adult language users understand, not words alone. We represent the source of speech not as a mouth or a body, but as a person. The logic that underlies everyday talk is the logic of human motivation.

This is precisely the logic that is missing in autism. Faces, facial movements, and associated sensory features such as vocal sounds are richly represented in the brains of normal infants and are therefore experientially meaningful. In normal children and adults, the cognitive pathways that elaborate representations of the qualities of people, such as mental states, are built on descriptions of faces, gestures, and voice intonations. But autistic individuals suffer from the congenital absence of a brain "organ" for person perception that would normally be constructed during their infancy and childhood. For them, the person percept is neither obligatory nor automatic, as it is for normal individuals. As a result, they do not speak the "language" of person and social order. We referred previously to brain regions that act as "editors" serving powerful social interests, regions that encourage the rest of the brain to report on features of the social environment. (The anatomy and evolutionary history of these regions will be spelled out in chapters 3 and 4.) Autistic children, I believe, lack a cognitive organ for person perception because their brains develop under the guidance of a dysfunctional editor.

Let us turn to the array of deficits seen in autism, discussing each in light of the proposed "dysfunctional editor." To begin with, autistic children pay little attention to one of the key building blocks for a perception of person—namely, faces. Their relative inattention to facial features was demonstrated by the following dramatic experiment.

Autistic and nonautistic children matched for mental age were given the task of sorting pictures of people who were shown from the shoulders up. The faces bore various expressions, and some of the pictured people wore hats. No instructions were given as to the basis for sorting the pictures. On the first try, the autistic children sorted the pictures according to the presence or absence of hats, whereas the nonautistic children sorted them according to facial expression. Without being given an evaluation of their efforts, the children were instructed, "Now, try it again a different way." On this second try, the autistic children sorted the pictures according to expression, and the nonautistic children sorted them according to hats. Taking both rounds of sorting together, it is clear that all the children could perceive and categorize both expression and hats. It is also clear that, left to themselves, and in comparison with the normal children, the autistic children did not find the facial expressions important.[16]

As we've seen, expressive faces and voices form the developmental building blocks that lead to the concept of person. The autistic child's inattentiveness to faces and voices causes initial impoverishment of representations of faces and their movements, and renders the child unable to construct the experience of other minds subsequently. Attributing a mind—replete with intentions, hopes, fears— to another is equivalent to attributing a subjective locus of experience. For autistic children, the understanding of others remains at the physical level rather than at the level of subjectivity. Indeed, deficits in understanding subjectivity have been demonstrated again and again in autistic children, as we will see.

Interestingly, autistic children are less attentive to the upper half of the face than are nonautistic children. The upper half of the face is of course dominated by the eyes and the expressive muscular activity around them. If advanced social representations depend on perceiving faces in the first instance, then they depend especially on perceiving the upper half of the face, because there are several kinds of social understanding mediated by the upper half of the face.

For one, direction of gaze is normally read as a signal of a subjective state (such as seeing, or thinking about). Although autistic children are able to use gaze direction to infer that someone is looking at something, they do not link gaze direction with the idea of someone's wishes or plans. It has been proposed therefore that autistic children fail to make the move from "looking at" to "thinking of." For another, patterns of muscle contraction around the eyes, including the forehead and eyebrows, are expressive. They are not the only indicators of feeling, but they are important for signaling dispositions. An inability to register these signals would leave one at a severe disadvantage in attributing subjective states to others. Finally, gaze direction, eye blinks, and eyebrow movements act as signals to structure conversation. Autistic individuals fail to employ or understand conversational pragmatics, the nonlinguistic acts that structure conversation as a cooperative social activity. In sum, both subjective states and conversational signals are normally read from the region of the eyes. A brain "editor" who did not pay attention to the eye region during infancy could cause subsequent defects in the ability to attribute mental states, to understand expressive communication, and to participate in conversations.[17]

We now turn from defects in attending to inputs such as faces, which are among the developmental prerequisites for understanding "person," to defects in the person concept itself. A primary manifestation of this defect is the inability to understand subjectivity. An interesting experiment revealed several aspects of the autistic child's deficits. Autistic children can use instrumental gestures, aimed at influencing the physical behavior of others, as can Down's syndrome and normal children. Such gestures include, for example, placing a finger in front of the mouth to signal "quiet" or beckoning with the hand to signal "come." But the experiment also revealed that, unlike the other two groups, these children do not use gestures that refer to a subjective state, such as patting another child in a consoling way, or putting one's hand before one's mouth to indicate embarrassment. In other words, although autistic children can use nonverbal gestures, they do so in ways that refer to physical states, but not in ways that refer to subjective states.[18]

In another experiment, high-functioning autistic children and normal children viewed five videotaped segments depicting children in different emotion-producing situations (for example, a boy loses his dog and is sad). The subjects were asked to label the protagonist's feelings, to report their own feelings, and to discuss the situations from the protagonists' perspectives. In the case of autistic children, the more intelligent children did better on these measures of empathy than the less intelligent ones. But intelligence did not seem to be a factor in the performance of the nonautistic children. The researchers suggest, therefore, that autistic children must use intellectual resources to decipher situations involving the subjective experiences of others, whereas normal children just "get it." As an analogy, imagine yourself back in math class, looking at an algebra equation. For some of us, understanding the equations required considerable effort; others seemed to look at the equations and just "get it." Researchers remark informally that autistic children understand emotional situations the way some of the

rest of us understand algebra—with effort. Another interesting finding among autistic children is their impaired ability to reflect on their
own and other people's minds as revealed by a paucity of words referring to cognitive states. Words like believe, dream, figure, pretend, and
wonder are rare in the spontaneous speech of autistic children.

Abnormalities in other aspects of language point to problems with
the concept of subjectivity. Strawson, whose writing on the philosophical concept of person was referred to at the beginning of the chapter,
emphasized that person predicates such as "in pain" or "depressed"
necessarily have *both* first-person and third-person uses. This is a
purely logical point, namely, that the notion of person implies both "I"
and "he/she" as loci of subjectivity. Although grammar and semantics
are used properly by autistic children, they fail to use personal pronouns correctly—for example, an autistic child may refer to herself as
"she" instead of "I."[19] Strawson's point receives empirical confirma-
tion in the syndrome of autism, once we view autism as a disorder in
which the very concept of subjectivity is lacking.

Autistic people are also notoriously poor conversationalists. To engage in conversation, one must be able to read and respond to a rapid
stream of paralinguistic signals, many involving the face. These signals
may be difficult for autistic individuals to register. But there is another
challenge as well: The concept of person and the activity of conversation are intimately related. The social psychologist Erving Goffman has
shown that in conversation interlocutors play with the notion of "self,"
using it in multiple ways and seeking public acknowledgment of it. As
we will see in chapter 6, conversation is where collaborative "person-
work" is carried out.[20] We need the person concept to "do" conversation, because this is the underlying *raison d'etre* of conversation. And
we need conversations as transient niches for the performances that
generate the social dimension of a person. Because autistic individuals
are missing the person concept, they cannot "do" conversation.

Do autistic children fail to develop a cognition of persons because
they have a dysfunctional, socially inattentive editor, or do they fail because they lack an editor *altogether*? Considering the autistic brain to
have been constructed under the guidance of a dysfunctional editor,
rather than under no editor at all, helps us to understand certain peculiarities. Autistic people may have intense preoccupations with, for example, the escalators in shopping malls, or bus routes, or the tactile
properties of sand. The devotion of a great deal of attention and repetition to narrow topics can result in savant capabilities, such as unusual
artistic or calculating abilities, a syndrome memorably depicted in the
movie *The Rainman*. Psychologist Uta Frith shows that the primary

problem in autism is neither peripheral sensory perception, attention, or the ability to categorize. Instead, the odd and seemingly narrow pre-occupations of autistic children prompt Frith to ask, "What stimuli will capture the attention of a person *who does not know what is worth attending to* [italics added]?" In other words, it is the focus of the autistic person's interests that appears to be awry. Whereas a typical school-age child is preoccupied with peer relationships, the inner re-portage of the autistic child may be taken up entirely with, for exam-ple, airline schedules. It is as though the editor, instead of sticking to the customary social agenda, became derailed onto an idiosyncratic *idée fixe*.[21]

But a failure to richly represent social elements could also follow from other kinds of processing problems. Just as an editor must have competent reporters racing to the main office with their reports from the field before he can select from them, an infant has to be able to at-tend to stimuli adequately in order to gather information, and the in-fant has to have a certain minimum of "reporters" covering various fronts. A brain unable to flexibly recruit attentional resources to events, especially events that change rapidly, would be analogous to a newspaper whose reporters could not manage to take notes in rapidly developing situations, and who thus would hand in gibberish or noth-ing at all to the editor. No enduring neural assemblies could be built and sustained under these conditions. Likewise, if visual reports were missing, a socially oriented editor might flounder for awhile, until she or he called on auditory reporters to increase their coverage so that the editor could promote a social agenda using only their reports. In fact, early in their development blind infants and children display "autistic-like features," but they do not go on to suffer from autism because of blindness.[22] This must be because blind children have the usual, so-cially inclined editor, which can direct its attention to other sensory re-ports, such as touch and sound, amplifying and elaborating these to develop the social representations of mind and motivation that nonautistic people share. A child who was sufficiently deprived in var-ious sensory domains, or sufficiently deprived of the expectable social environment from which it would normally gather experience, would be expected to develop autistically, even though structures of the child's brain might possess the normal inclinations to attend to social experiences.

The experiments we have looked at support my proposal that a dys-functional editor is at work in the young autistic brain, depriving it of the building blocks from which the person concept can ultimately be built. Whether for peripheral "information-gathering" reasons, or more central "editing" reasons, autistic children are pulled off the track that normal children follow. For autistic children, faces and related social features have not "grabbed control of the media." Consequently, the neural assemblies that encode the appearances and activities of others are left sparse and recessive, the primary basis for developing more advanced descriptions of social events is absent, and percepts involving subjectivity are as unavailable as is the color red to a color-blind person. (Parallel arguments apply to voices and to social touch, which ultimately would be expected to become linked with vision in social representations.) Thus, the "language" of both a person concept and the social order, which normally develops from innate mechanisms, is absent in autistic children.

In this chapter, we focused on dimension of the concept of person—on how subjectivity comes to be attributed to bodies. We reviewed two general syndromes in which there are deficits in attributing mind to others or oneself. The first was a group of syndromes involving acquired brain damage, the misidentification syndromes. The second was a syndrome that, when it occurs, is present from birth—autism. We discussed the brain basis of misidentification syndromes, but the brain basis of autism was only hinted at, by reference to an "editor." The nature of the editor will occupy us in more detail in chapters 3 and 4.

2

Building the Experience of Mind

Theory of Mind in Children

It is one thing to notice someone's bodily movements or gestures and quite another to attribute a mental state to him or her. For attributing a mental state—such as a wish, an intention, or a belief—requires us to free ourselves from the world of things as they are. When we think of someone having a belief that is incorrect or a mental picture of an imaginary state of affairs, our thought stands free from material facts. In this chapter, we gather more clues about how and why we attribute mental states to people. The clues come from our knowledge of normal development, from informed guesses about the evolutionary history of our species, and from a careful analysis of developmental disorders such as autism.

One might think that human babies and children would have the ability to attribute beliefs to others from the time they begin to speak. But this is not the case, as developmental psychologists have demonstrated. To test children's abilities to conceptualize the beliefs of others in the presence of a contradicting reality, researchers ask children to watch a play or listen to a story of the following general form: "Here are John and Terry. Now see them opening a box and putting a candy inside it. Oh, someone is calling to John to go outside. Away he goes. Now Terry is all alone. Look, Terry is taking the candy from the box, and he is putting it behind the curtain. Now Terry is waiting for John to come back. Here comes John, back in the room. John wants the candy! *Experimenter to child:* Where will John go to look for the candy?"

Typically, children under the age of 4 will answer, erroneously, "Behind the curtain," indicating they do not distinguish between their own knowledge and that of the character John, who was absent when the candy was placed behind the curtain. Slightly more than half the children in the 4- to 6-year-old range are able to answer correctly— namely, that John will look for the candy in the box. Most children over the age of 6 answer correctly.

A simpler version of this test is the "Smarties" test. Smarties are a type of candy familiar to English children, which come in a character- istic long, thin package. A Smarties package is shown to a child, who is asked, "What is in here?" The child answers, "Smarties." The pack- age is then opened, and the child learns that the package contains pencils, not Smarties. The package is closed again, and a new person enters the room. "Here is Tom," says the experimenter. The experi- menter asks the child, "We will show Tom this package. What will Tom think is in the package?" Again, children under 4 answer incor- rectly, "Pencils," showing their inability to attribute a false belief to another person.

Such results raise an important question. A belief can be thought of as being like a picture—that is, a representation somehow "in the head." Researchers asked themselves, do young children have diffi- culty understanding representations in general, or understanding men- tal ones only? An experiment that used a camera answered this question quite simply. In it, children were taught to use a Polaroid camera. They used the camera to take a picture of an object in one lo- cation. Then, while the picture was developing, the children watched as the object was moved to a new location. Before the picture came out, they were asked to say where the object would be *in the picture.* Again, children under 4 erroneously predicted the photograph would show the scene as it currently lay before them, rather than as it was when they photographed it. Their responses suggested that they had trouble distinguishing representations of any kind—photographic or mental—from reality.

A possible interpretation of all these findings is that young children hold to a strong default assumption—namely, that beliefs and images correspond to reality. This interpretation is given weight by the fact that redesigning the experiment to reduce the emphasis on the reality, or to increase the emphasis on the representation, allows 3-year-olds to pass the "false belief" test. For example, in one experiment, children were allowed to participate by "being tricky" and changing an object's location in order to deceive an absent person. This maneuver height- ens the emphasis on the false belief, compared to the John–Terry and the Smarties experiments. Under these conditions, 3-year-olds are able to ascribe a false belief. [1]

Could there be a difference, though, in the way our brains handle nonmental representations, such as photographs or maps, and mental representations, such as false beliefs? Despite the fact that normal children fail at both when they are younger and succeed at both later on, there is indeed evidence that these skills depend on different mechanisms. The representational skills that have to do specifically with mental representation are called "theory of mind." Shortly we will look at autistic children again, who are able to understand mechanical representations such as photographs, but not *mental* representations. First, however, let us look at the evolutionary history of "theory of mind."

Theory of Mind in Apes and Monkeys

To understand how we came to be as we are, researchers sometimes look for clues in the similarities and differences between ourselves and our primate relatives. What about apes and monkeys? Are they able to represent others as having knowledge different from their own? Whether any nonhuman primate truly attributes belief to another has been difficult to establish. Many observations that might at first give the appearance of an animal manipulating another's direction of attention could also be interpreted more conservatively—for example, as the chance combination of noninsightful behaviors. There have been two approaches to the question of whether monkeys and apes possess a theory of mind. One is the collection of observations from field primatologists. Naturalistic observations have been systematically collected; this is one of several examples.

> The following account was contributed to our corpus by Kummer: it concerns Hamadryas baboons, in which one large "leader" male typically has long-term exclusive mating and social interactions with several females, but in which the latter can occasionally contrive interactions with other males. Kummer observed a female spend 20 minutes moving into a position where she could groom a subadult male, an action which would not be tolerated if witnessed by her leader male. What is important is that she adjusted her position carefully such that the leader male could see the top part of her, but not the young male, nor the female's hands which were surreptitiously grooming him.[2]

From this observation, the authors concluded that the female was able to understand the male leader's view, even though it was different from her own. Her behavior showed she was able to imagine the male's representation of the world, and thus that she had a theory of mind. And other reports have suggested that apes in the wild employ deception to manipulate the attention of other animals so that they can achieve their own ends without interference.

A second approach to discovering whether nonhuman primates understand others' mental lives is to test them using experimental methods designed to rule out competing explanations for their behavior. Imaginative experiments have been carried out using captive and free-ranging vervet monkeys, and captive chimpanzees. Vervet monkeys' ability to represent the minds of other vervets is not impressive. The evidence from captive chimpanzees is somewhat more convincing, however, as the following experiment shows. Two boxes were placed before juvenile chimpanzees. Food was placed by an experimenter in one of the two boxes, but this was done while a screen was placed between the boxes and the chimpanzees, so that they could not see in which box the food was placed. Standing by were two other experimenters. One was positioned so that he could see the boxes as they were being baited—and the chimpanzees could see that he could see. The other was placed so that the experimenter could see no more than the animals themselves. After one of the boxes was baited, the screen was removed. The chimpanzees were given only one opportunity to select the correct box, so their lack of direct knowledge was a handicap. Yet they were able, by pulling a string, to "choose" one of the two experimenters who were standing by. The chosen experimenter would tap one of the boxes. The animal could then make its choice, using the "advice" of the experimenter if it wished. Of four animals tested, three chose the knowledgeable experimenter more often than the ignorant one, seeming to indicate that they understood both "seeing" and "knowing," which are mental states. But one of the three animals did not follow the advice of the knowledgeable experimenter after she received it. Thus, only two of the four animals could be said to have fully solved the problem.

In interpreting these results, we have to bear in mind that what extensively domesticated chimpanzees can do in a laboratory probably differs considerably from what their wild counterparts would normally do under natural conditions, where the tasks and the events are quite different. As we have just seen, in laboratory demonstrations such as the food-in-the-box experiment, the results are mixed. Indeed, the eminent primatologist David Premack believes the evidence for theory of mind in any nonhuman primate is inconclusive and made the commonsense observation that a chimpanzee cannot attribute a mental state to others that it does not have itself. According to Premack, it's not likely an ape can attribute anything more sophisticated than seeing, wanting, and expecting, which are the simple mental states that chimpanzees themselves possess. Whatever the chimpanzee's theory of mind, Premack concluded, it is likely to be much weaker and less elaborate than the human one.³

Although the phrase "theory of mind" seems to imply that we are studying a unitary phenomenon, there may be many ways in which animals evaluate the behavior of other animals, depending on the context, the species, and individual experience. Accounts from natural settings, such as that of the female baboon carefully grooming the young male out of the sight of the group's leader, strongly suggest that wild apes have at least some version of a theory of mind, but scientists have yet to understand all the ecological variables involved in this sort of behavior.

Constructing Mind—A Human Specialization

The issue of theory of mind has captured the attention of both primatologists and developmental psychologists. It has been proposed that theory of mind is but one aspect of primate "social intelligence," a cognitive specialization selectively encouraged by nature. This specialization may even be relatively isolated from the monkey's other capabilities, for it has been shown that although monkeys appear to think logically in a social setting, drawing appropriate conclusions from one another's behavior, they cannot solve analogous logical problems with inanimate objects in the laboratory.

Why would theory of mind cognition have been particularly advantageous in our evolutionary past? Primates evolved to live in ever-more-complex social groups, and to use rapid and sensitive means of signaling—namely, visually perceived gestures and vocalizations—as opposed to scent. (The brain changes that accompanied this trend are examined in detail in chapter 4.) As visual and auditory signaling became ever-more differentiated, and social groups more complex, the primate's ability to perceive and respond to social signals must have been challenged to keep pace. The psychologist Nicholas Humphrey pointed out that when individuals become competent at reading others' intentions, evolutionary pressure on the capacity to deceive is increased, leading to greater challenges to the capacity to read others. That is, the presence of individuals who have great social competence "heats up" selection pressure in a way that environmental demands external to the animals themselves do not. This situation forces a specialization to develop in relative isolation from other competences, just as an organ can evolve independently of other organs. The presence of socially selective neurons in macaque monkey brains, it has been argued, reflects the operation of evolutionary pressure to develop just such a specifically social intelligence.[4] (We shall learn more about these neurons in the next chapter.)

In addition to evolutionary plausibility, there are other arguments for the existence of a relative specialization in the brain's processing of certain kinds of information. For example, in humans, cognition whose subject matter is other minds operates on a different set of inputs from cognition that relates, for example, to music or mathematics. Furthermore, aspects of social cognition can be selectively absent, as we saw in the last chapter. Although children with autism have a number of symptoms, the core diagnostic criterion is impairment in social communication. Because some autistic individuals are otherwise normal in their cognitive abilities, it is reasonable to think there is a specialized neural system that is selectively damaged in these individuals.

Conversely, a rare disorder called Williams syndrome seems to selectively spare aspects of social cognition. Williams syndrome is a genetically caused disorder that can be diagnosed at birth from a characteristic set of physical findings including facial appearance and cardiac abnormalities. An underlying problem in calcium metabolism, critical for regulating many physical processes, is thought to be the cause of faulty development in both the bodies and the brains of children with the disorder. Although children with Williams syndrome usually have low intelligence quotients (IQs) and are unable to perform a wide variety of cognitive tasks, aspects of their use of language are quite advanced, they do much better than matched controls at recognizing faces, and they are far superior to autistic children at theory-of-mind tasks—even when compared with autistic children whose IQs are much higher than their own.[5]

Thus, researchers are beginning to understand how we construct a concept of mind by studying individuals in whom mind-making systems seem either to have been selectively damaged—as in autism—or selectively spared, as in Williams syndrome. Although Williams syndrome has only come to be studied in detail by psychologists in recent years, research on autism has a longer history. There has been time for competing theories about the central cognitive failure in autism to crystallize. What are these theories?

According to one idea, autistic persons have a primary defect in theory of mind. Recall that theory of mind allows us to imagine the mental states of others—to attribute beliefs, goals, and desires. We saw that normal children become able to attribute knowledge to others beginning around age 4—earlier, if deception is emphasized. Significantly, the ability to understand false belief in another person eludes the autistic child until much later, if he or she indeed achieves it at all. Although autistic children with mental ages of 4 years fail false-belief tasks, they do *better* than normal children on the Polaroid task described above. That is, they correctly state what the photograph will show, even though it is different from the reality they know to be true. This shows that the autistic child's trouble in understanding false belief is not the result of a generalized problem in understanding representations. Rather, it indicates that their difficulty is restricted to conceptualizing human mental states.[6]

A competing idea is that these children lack normal emotions that bind us to other human beings. Indeed, it had struck Kanner that autistic children seemed to possess "an innate inability to form the usual, biologically provided affective contact with people." Along these lines, the psychiatrist R. Peter Hobson theorizes that autistic children lack what is necessary for reciprocal, emotionally charged personal relations with other people. This hypothesized deficit would have several consequences. One is that autistic children would not grasp the idea of other minds; another is that they would not grasp the many different social constructions that may be placed on the world by persons with their various orientations. This in turn would prevent the ability to think flexibly and to pretend. Impairments in autistic children's understanding of emotional expression, their lack of interest in facial expressions of emotion, their lack of response to distress in others, and their difficulty understanding emotional situations involving others all support, but do not prove, Hobson's theory.[7]

These competing explanations of autism were already in place when scientists' attention began to be drawn to some important findings in the brains of monkeys—namely, that socially responsive single neurons were being discovered in areas of the brain traditionally associated with emotion. This led to the idea that perhaps these brain areas, instead of being dedicated to emotion, were specialized for processing others' social intentions. According to the theory, the attribution of intentions and dispositions to others would reflect the operation of a brain mechanism that had evolved to respond to significant gestures and expressions. A malfunctioning of this "social module" could explain the deficits in autism. The dichotomy between "cold" social cognition— the attribution of belief—and "hot" social cognition—emotional relatedness—was replaced by the idea of a single brain system specialized for responding to social signals of all kinds, a system that would ultimately construct representations of mind.[8]

The basic principle underlying this brain system is straightforward. Monkeys, apes, and humans must all gear their behavior to that of the other members of the group in which they live. Because primate social groups are complex, social responses are very diverse, comprising such behavior as submissive deference, jealous assertion, maternal protectiveness, macho exhibitionism, affiliative approach, running away, courtship behavior, appeals for help, and so on. Second, social responses are exquisitely responsive to the current social situation, a constantly fluctuating scene involving mates and potential mates, offspring, allies, rivals, bullies, in-groups, and so on. This scene is the environment of evolutionary adaptedness, shaping cognitive processes in primates and humankind. What the discovery of socially responsive neurons revealed is that the primate brain evolved a specialized system for producing mutually regulated behavior in these complex social environments.

It works like this. I perceive a gesture or expression on the part of another individual, in a particular context generated either by our own past history, or by the presence of other individuals—a context that could be one of rivalry, let's say, or romance. The gesture of the other individual is encoded by areas of my brain that index it by automatically linking it to the appropriate response: The perception of someone trying to take from me something I want causes my heart rate to increase, and my muscles to prepare for an assertive action; the perception of someone flirting evokes a different pattern of heart rate and blood-flow changes and causes me to increase or decrease eye contact. In other words, current social inputs are mapped onto an innate "alphabet" in the brain consisting of representations of social situations prewired to an appropriate response. As a result of this wiring, the passage from social perception to bodily reaction is not carefully planned and willed. Instead, it is the automatic product of a long evolutionary history in which individuals have had to compete, reproduce, and care for their young—all while integrating themselves into groups of other individuals similarly engaged. An individual's intention is encoded by the response it evokes in the perceiver. In other words, I know someone is flirting by the changes the person's behavior evokes in me. Although that individual's intentions are being registered, a picture of his or her "mind" is still not necessary in order for there to be a response.

Chimpanzees and baboons compete with one another, flirt with one another, appease one another. But the transition to constructing mind takes us beyond the common social heritage we share with our primate relatives. A great cognitive divide separated us from our nonhuman ancestors and separates us today from our nonhuman counterparts. At some period in our evolutionary past, as a result of our brains evolving in a highly social environment, humans added a conceptual level to the percept of a fellow being—mind. Perhaps evolution provided an impetus, as Machiavellian intelligence theory proposes, through the spiraling effects of deception and counterdeception. Alternatively, consider the fact that many gestures are ambiguous in their import. The increasing load of complex and shifting social signals that our ancestors were beginning to process might have led to paralysis—to breakdown in the capacity to respond—unless a way could be found to organize it all. The ability to construct a concept of mind offers a solution to this problem: The advantage of the concept of person is that it rapidly, automatically organizes the sights and sounds of other individuals.[9] And through its tie to a social order, it provides us with a new system for gearing our actions into those of our neighbors, a system defined by shoulds and oughts rather than by snarls and grimaces. This new way of perceiving the sights and sounds of our fellow humans is the basis of our theory of mind.

Children become members of the social order gradually. Not only must they learn the rules of their particular culture, but they must learn how to attach social qualities to persons, things like status and moral qualities, for these are arbitrary rather than intrinsic to human bodies. Here is where a remarkable feature of children's behavior comes in—their devotion to pretend play. Pretense allows the child to provisionally characterize an object in a way that is at odds with its appearance (as when pretending a banana is a telephone), or to collaborate with others in taking on temporary roles (as in playing school or house). By practicing the assignment of arbitrary rules and characteristics, and requiring themselves to act "as if" those are real, children practice participating in the social order. Once again, this brings us to autism, for one of the distinguishing features of the disorder is that autistic children do not pretend. Normal pretend play, then, reflects the immature operation of the person concept; a concept of mind and the ability to integrate oneself into the social order reflect its mature operation.[10]

There is experimental evidence showing that we link the perception of bodily features with the social order by the intervening concept of mental characteristics. Subjects in a psychology experiment were given a large set of unknown photographed faces to look at. For some faces, they were asked to make judgments about personality, and for others, judgments about visual features of the face. Later, they were presented with these faces, mixed in with a larger set they had not seen. Their recall of the "target" faces was better when they had made judgments about personality characteristics than when they had made judgments about physical features.[11] This result is typical of the improvement in cognitive processing, which occurs when "semantic" as opposed to "featural" encoding takes place. Just as nonsense words are hard to recall because no semantic encoding occurs, faces are hard to recall unless mind and a place in the social order are assigned to them. Extensive research on memory for faces led the psychologist Vicki Bruce to conclude,

> It seems that face perception invokes attributional processes which go far beyond the information given. Shown only a face, we are prepared to judge a person's emotional state, personality traits, probable employment, and possible fate.
>
> Instructing subjects to form personality impressions from faces (the "trait" condition) is likely to maximize visually derived semantic coding.[12]

In conclusion, we have examined how the concept of mind is developed by children as they mature and have speculated as to how and why it was developed by our species in its evolutionary history. Sometime after the divergence between humans and other primates, it appears that our ancestors took off on an evolutionary trajectory leading from extensive sociality to theory of mind and the concept of person. Their socially responsive brains evolved to yield new high-level descriptions linked with a social order—descriptions of mind and person. Like the bones of the reptilian jaw, socially selective neural ensembles in primates were rearranged to produce something new.

3

The Brain's Social Specialization

Momentous Discoveries

I have been referring to brain structures that allow us to attribute mind to bodies. I even suggested that the brain has an "editor" that encourages the recording of social features during infancy, inscribing them preferentially onto the hardware of the developing human brain. Where are these brain structures, and how do they work together to produce such remarkable effects? In this chapter, we begin to look at the "social brain" and how its secrets were unlocked by scientists working in places as varied as brain research laboratories and African jungles.

To understand their discoveries, we need to map out a few key landmarks of the primate brain.[1] Figure 1.1 depicted a human brain shown both from the outside, and from the medial side (which is like the cut surface of an apple when it is cut in half). The outer layer of the brain is called the cortex. The major components of the brain, going from back to front, are the occipital, parietal, temporal, and frontal lobes, which are paired, one in each hemisphere. Deep within the temporal lobe is a cluster of neurons called the amygdala, a nut-sized structure traditionally believed to be important in emotion. The hippocampus, also found within the temporal lobe, is classically associated with memory processes. The cortex lining the base of the frontal lobe, the part that lies above the sockets of the eyes, is called the orbital frontal cortex. A cortical region found on the medial surface of each hemisphere, which protrudes at its front, or anterior, end into the frontal lobe, is called the cingulate gyrus. Like the amygdala, the orbital frontal and anterior cingulate cortices have often been linked to emotional processes.

But, as we see in this chapter, researchers are beginning to understand them differently—in the context of social cognition rather than emotion.

In the 1950s, researchers discovered that neurons in certain regions of the brain respond in specific ways to visual stimulation. Responses to small moving dots, for example, were first shown in neurons of the retina, a sheet that lines the back of the eye and that is the initial receiving station for visual information coming from the outside world.[2] The pioneering vision researcher David Hubel extended this research by following the eyes' pathways into the brain itself. First, he studied a region called the lateral geniculate nucleus, which receives inputs from the retina. Then he moved to the striate cortex, an area at the back of the brain that is the next waystation for incoming visual information. Understanding the visual cortex was a reasonable place to start in the quest for understanding how the brain makes sense of the world around it, and the study of visual processes has indeed been productive. In groundbreaking work, Hubel and his colleague, Torsten Wiesel, showed that striate neurons in cats responded to very specific aspects of the animal's visual experience. Recording from neurons one at a time, they showed that single neurons could be activated by particular features of the visual environment—lines shown at particular angles, or light–dark boundaries. They suggested that the activity of hundreds of thousands of such neurons, each with its own sensitivity to simple visual features, might combine to yield a perception of complex objects and the integrated experience of our visual world with which we are familiar.

Now we come to a key event. Up until this point, neuroscientists had treated minds and brains as if they were socially isolated, like shipwrecked Robinson Crusoes. The developments we are about to trace, however, echo the episode in which Crusoe discovered he was not alone. Readers will recall the fateful moment in which the shipwrecked sailor, after years of solitude, encountered a mark on the sand: "It happened one day about noon going towards my boat, I was exceedingly surprised with the print of a man's naked foot on the shore, which was very plain to be seen in the sand. I stood like one thunder-struck, or as if I had seen an apparition."[3]

In the case of the brain, the portentous mark of sociality was discovered by a visual neurophysiologist, Charles Gross. In the 1960s, Gross undertook to extend Hubel and Wiesel's techniques to other brain regions. Unlike most researchers, however, he decided not to work near the margins of brain territory that had already been explored. Instead, he moved into an area that receives neural inputs from primary visual cortex through several intermediate steps. This area, the inferotemporal cortex, was suspected of being part of the visual system, but its specific characteristics had not been studied in detail. Gross wanted to map the visual receptive fields of single neurons, and test their sensitivity to features of visual stimuli.

The basic technique of recording from single neurons in monkeys was pioneered by the physiologist Edward Evarts and is technically quite demanding. The researcher's aim is to bring very fine-tipped electrodes into contact with individual neurons in the brain. He or she begins by placing a monkey in a comfortable position in a specially designed chair. A carefully designed opening in the skull, made in an earlier surgical procedure, is uncapped. Through it a recording electrode is lowered and passed into the brain, micrometer by micrometer. Fine wires attached to the outside end of the electrode conduct the electrical signals from single neurons to a series of amplifiers and recording equipment. Such equipment allowed Gross and his co-workers to see and hear neurons in the inferotemporal cortex, and to make a permanent record of their activity. Even an alert animal cannot feel an electrode passing through its brain, because the brain contains no sensory nerve endings, unlike the skin and other parts of the body. But Gross's monkey was fully anesthetized. Not only was the animal unaware of the electrode, but the medication ensured that its eyes would not change position, a precaution that is critical when the goal is to map the visual field in front of the animal onto activity in vision-related regions of the brain. By keeping the monkey's eyes open while it "slept," the researchers could activate its retina and the visual regions of the brain by projecting visual stimuli on a screen in front of it.

To this already challenging experiment, Gross and his co-workers added demanding testing conditions. For each neuron in inferotemporal cortex that they isolated with their recording electrodes, they tested responses both to the locations of stimuli in the visual field, and to visual features such as shape, color, and movement. The results they obtained were of great significance. In a key 1972 article, they reported that some cells responded best to specific, complex stimuli, such as dark shapes that the experimenters cut out and moved about on a lighted screen before the monkey subjects. They went on to describe these stimuli, one series in particular:

> The most common dark stimuli used were a variety of rectangles or slits . . . and the shadow of a human or monkey hand. The use of the latter stimuli was begun one day when, having failed to drive a unit with any light stimulus, we waved a hand at the stimulus screen and elicited a very vigorous response from the previously unresponsive neuron. We

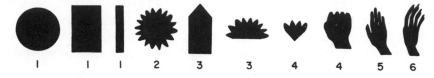

Figure 3.1 Examples of cutout shapes which Gross and colleagues used to test the "hand" cell. The stimuli are arranged from left to right in order of increasing ability to drive the neuron from none (1) or little (2 and 3) to maximum (6). [Figure from "Visual properties of neurons in inferotemporal cortex of the macaque" by C. Gross, C. Rocha-Miranda, and D. Bender, (1972). *Journal of Neurophysiology*, 35, p. 104. Reproduced by permission of the American Physiological Society.]

> then spent the next 12 hr testing various paper cutouts in an attempt to find the trigger feature for this unit. When the entire set of stimuli used were ranked according to the strength of the response that they produced, we could not find a simple physical dimension that correlated with this rank order. However, the rank order of adequate stimuli did correlate with similarity (for us) to the shadow of a monkey hand. The relative adequacy of a few of these stimuli is shown in Fig. 6 [presented as Figure 3.1 here]. Curiously, fingers pointing downward elicited very little response as compared to fingers pointing upward or laterally, the usual orientations in which the animal would see its own hand.[4]

Until this moment, researchers had relied exclusively on geometric, nonsocial stimuli, such as dark rectangles, slanted lines, or moving dots, to study the visual system. Gross and his students were the first to describe a neuron activated specifically by a bodily feature. Although the report also mentioned a few cells that responded to faces, these cells were relatively ignored by the researchers, whereas the hand-responsive cell received much attention. This is understandable, as the face-responsive cells were not systematically studied in that initial experiment, whereas the "hand" cell clearly was—for 12 hours!

These observations appeared to lend support to a theory widely held at the time. The theory said that cells in the primary visual cortex (the cells studied by Hubel and Wiesel) encoded very elemental visual features, such as light–dark boundaries and short line segments. These cells sent information, via electrical activity communicated from neuron to neuron, "downstream" to other brain regions. Electrical activity from two such simple cells might converge on a third: Thus, coding for various kinds of simple features would converge, giving rise to cells that responded to complex combinations of features. These, in turn, would feed to other cells whose responses to complex objects would be still more specific. For example, the bookcase before me presents a large number of lines, both vertical and horizontal, many areas in which there are light–dark boundaries, and a few textured surfaces. Let's assume there are individual cells in my visual cortex that fire when presented with vertical lines at specific locations, others that fire when presented with horizontal lines, others that fire in response to light–dark boundaries, and so on. When these cells are activated, they transmit their activity in turn to still other cells, where the activity is combined. The recipient cells, then, fire in response to a combination of features, such as a wood-grain texture bounded by horizontal light–dark boundaries. The outputs of these cells might converge on still other cells, so that ultimately my brain would have cells that respond specifically to the combination of features that make up my bookcase. The "hand cell" was believed to illustrate just this kind of convergence.

In the years following Gross's discovery, this simple, hierarchical theory of vision did not hold up as an accurate explanation for how our brains process the visual world. The idea that there might be a neuron for each specific object we come across in the world was facetiously called the "grandmother cell" theory, for it predicted that our brain would contain a neuron that would fire only on seeing our grandmother! Today, researchers accept that some visual encoding is carried out by small clusters of neurons very sensitive to particular features of our environment. But equally important, researchers have continued to find many kinds of neurons, each responding to some very simple feature in the visual field. They believe that neurons work collectively: The encoding of complex objects occurs not in a few cells at the top of a processing pyramid, but through the joint, temporally coordinated activity of millions of neurons together.[5] This ability of our brain, called parallel distributed encoding, became a dominant theory a few years after Gross's work was reported. Parallel distributed processing gave scientists a way to understand the integrated view we have of our world, but it didn't explain how an individual cell could be very specific in its responses to a complex object. Neurons that responded to a handlike shape or a face could not be understood within this new distributed view of the brain. For this reason, and because such experiments are very difficult to carry out, Gross's findings unfortunately were not pursued vigorously.

It was almost 10 years later, in 1981, that Gross, this time with Robert Desimone and Charles Bruce, published a systematic study of cells that responded specifically to faces in the nearby superior temporal sulcus. The superior temporal sulcus is a prominent landmark in the temporal lobes of nonhuman primates and may be clearly seen in human brains as well. In this study of monkey neurons, Gross and his colleagues documented another serendipitous observation—namely, that for 15 of the cells studied, the best stimulus was the sight of a person walking:

> Informal observations suggested that the pattern of movement generated by walking and not the person per se was crucial for the response of these units. For example, a person seated in a moving chair or a person walking with the lower part of the body shielded elicited little or no response from these units. Large inanimate moving objects also elicited little or no response. . . . Furthermore, some of these units gave discrete responses to each step of a person's movement. Half of these units responded preferentially to particular directions of walking.[6]

The significance and role of these neurons, which were responsive to a specific kind of movement by persons but not movement of inanimate objects, were not further pursued by these researchers. Together with evidence for responsiveness to hands and faces, however, the finding provided another hint that there are neurons in the primate brain that are quite specialized for social features of the environment.

Socially responsive cells have not only appeared in the work of vision researchers. They also turned up in studies of emotion. Edmund Rolls of Oxford University has long been concerned with brain mechanisms of learning, especially how learning is affected by rewarding or aversive experiences. The goal of one of Rolls's studies was to understand how motivation affects the objects we perceive. Thinking that the amygdala might form an intermediate link in associating the positive or negative aspects of an object with its visual appearance, Rolls and his co-workers set out to record neurons in the amygdala, while presenting monkeys with rewarding stimuli such as food, and a variety of aversive stimuli such as the taste of salty water, puffs of air on the animal's face, and significantly, a threatening facial expression that Rolls himself made at the animal subject. In reporting the results of their study, the authors noted somewhat parenthetically that nine of the neurons that were visually sensitive responded best to faces or to pictures of faces, and that two other neurons were inhibited only by faces and not other visual stimuli. Apparently these neurons did not respond to aversive stimuli, such as the salty water, but were specifically responsive to the sight of faces. Faces had been used merely as one of the aversive stimuli, but it became clear during the experiment that they are significant in their own right.[7]

Although Gross's and Rolls's observations were accidental and have been viewed as controversial because they suggest a "grandmother cell" interpretation, they have proved beyond any doubt that some neurons respond preferentially and selectively to social aspects of our world. Building on their results, other researchers have begun to show how the brain assembles these responses into coherent descriptions of the social environment.

Constructing Social Descriptions in the Brain

Studies of socially responsive neurons in monkeys have been carried out primarily in the superior temporal sulcus, the inferotemporal cortex, and the amygdala and nearby cortex. Only a minority of neurons in these regions respond specifically to social stimuli. For example, Desimone and his colleagues systematically studied 151 neurons in the inferotemporal cortex. Of these, 110 gave sufficiently strong and consistent responses to allow further analysis: Testing showed 66 were responsive to some stimuli but not to others—that is, they were to some degree selective—and a total of only five neurons were selective for specific objects, two for hands, and three for faces. By moving into the superior temporal sulcus, however, where face-selective cells had been found previously, they were able to locate a small zone where such cells could be found consistently. In this zone, 17 of the 50 cells studied responded more strongly to faces than to other complex objects. Similarly, in the amygdala as a whole, only about 10% or less of neurons tested are socially responsive; however, these are concentrated in certain subregions.[8]

It is not unusual to find a low percentage of specifically responsive cells in brain areas such as these, which are not primary sensory or motor regions. Why this is so is a matter of speculation. One reasonable theory is that these neurons link, by reciprocal connections, networks of cells distributed throughout sensory cortices. Such linking neurons would be triggered only when specific neural combinations are activated in more primary sensory regions. Although this idea has some resemblance to the "grandmother cell" theory of representation, it is different in that the coding is not carried out by the linking cell alone, but rather by all the cells that are simultaneously activated.[9] Thus, neurons in regions like the superior temporal sulcus and amygdala might only be triggered by very specific social stimuli, whose features are encoded in cortical activity elsewhere.

Numerous or rare, it still had to be proven that "face" cells were what they seemed to be. Scientists, skeptical by nature, wanted to determine to what extent "face" cells were indeed selective only for faces and not for other complex objects. Researchers presented animals with a large variety of objects, as well as pictures of faces, to ascertain how selective the neurons were for faces. They discovered that some populations of cells are selective for, but are not dedicated only to faces; this became evident because the cells responded weakly to other visual stimuli as well.[10] But a population of cells that was highly selective for human and monkey faces, in contrast to all other complex objects, was found deep within the superior temporal sulcus.

Could the cells really be responding to some incidental visual feature (a line or dark–light boundary, for example) that just happened to be in the face? Because the neurons responded to faces regardless of changes in color, size, distance, position within the visual field, or orientation (degree of tilt) of the face, this explanation became increasingly unlikely. In addition, when pictures of faces were scrambled, so that all features were still present, but jumbled so as to make the face unrecognizable as a face, the response disappeared. Taken together, these studies provided good evidence that there are cells which respond preferentially to faces and that the response is not just to some incidental visual feature contained within the picture.

Recently, Edmund Rolls's group, in collaboration with the vision scientist Vilayanur Ramachandran, have demonstrated conclusively that the cells are responding to "faceness" as opposed to incidental visual features in the face picture. The design of their study was based on some interesting facts about visual perception in general. Objects depicted in high-contrast, black-and-white photographs are often difficult to recognize because we need various degrees of shading to help us perceive shape. If we are first shown a photograph of an object that is recognizable because it contains the normal amount of gray shading, however, followed by a high-contrast version of the photograph, we become able to "see" the object in the high-contrast version. This means that the same high-contrast picture may look either like a jumble of dark shapes, or like a recognizable object, depending on whether the viewer's brain has been "trained" to see the object by previous exposure to a more conventional picture of it.

Rolls's group showed high-contrast pictures of faces to monkeys, exploiting the fact that the perception of a face is only possible if grayscale pictures are shown first. Single neurons in the superior temporal sulcus and inferotemporal cortex of the monkeys did not respond to the high-contrast images of faces when these were shown first; they did respond to these images when they were shown *after* the animal had seen the gray-scale version. These results provide very convincing evidence that temporal lobe neurons are sensitive to the percept of a face, and not to some incidental visual feature of the face picture.[11]

But perhaps the neurons that were responsive to faces were really sensitive to any emotionally charged stimulus. To answer this possibility, experimenters have shown that cells respond to a face just as strongly the fifth or sixth time it is presented as they do the first time. Because emotional impact should decrease with repetition, these findings rule against a simple explanation based on emotional arousal. Moreover, these cells did not respond to other stimuli known to be emotionally significant to monkeys, such as the sight of snakes or syringes.

Monkeys almost always live in complex social groups. So do human beings. But we are not unique in being social—so are wolves, dolphins, elephants, and ants. Other species also must have mechanisms for responding to social cues, mechanisms unique to their evolutionary histories. What researchers who study primate brains want to know is, what brain mechanisms do *primates* use? The presence of specialized brain responses to social features suggests that human social behavior, like that of our primate relatives, has a neural basis we can study and come to understand. It is only once we have understood the details of our particular kind of social processing, by using information from monkeys and—as we will do in later chapters—combining that knowledge with studies of the human brain, that we will be in a position to understand how human social cognition sets us apart from other social species.

To this end we have already reviewed the discovery and characterization of socially responsive neurons in monkeys in great detail. But how are the bits and pieces of the outside social world assembled in the primate brain, to produce integrated perceptions of meaningful social events? How do our brains tell the difference between someone approaching with friendly intent and someone whose aims are hostile? To start with, we can assume that the visual features of a face have to be put together to yield an image of a particular individual who has a unique identity—*who* is approaching gives us access to our past interactions with this individual. Next, we need to be able to put together bits of movement that we see around someone's eyes and mouth to get an integrated impression of the person's disposition. Finally, our brain would need to use information from head position and body movement to form a description of where this person is looking or going. In short, our brains must combine information regarding the motions, positions, and identities of the people around us to come up with descriptions of their social intentions.

In fact, some neurons that are sensitive to faces respond best to particular features of the face or to the spatial relations of features within the face, such as the distance between the eyes and the mouth. Such neurons might be particularly useful for distinguishing different faces from one another. Indeed, researchers found that a monkey's neurons responded differently to pictures of different individuals. We now believe that even a small population of face-selective neurons, taken as a whole, may carry enough information to identify individual faces: some populations of face-responsive cells carry information regarding physical characteristics of faces, whereas others carry information regarding familiarity.[12]

Aside from facial features, facial expressions can be very important in signaling the dispositions and intentions of other animals.[13] Cells sensitive to facial expression found in the superior temporal sulcus respond to the same expression in both humans and monkeys. And the cells that fire on seeing the "threat" faces of a monkey, which involves opening of the mouth, do not respond to mouth opening that occurs during chewing or other expressions. So the cell's response is not caused by an incidental visual feature—the open mouth—but to the meaningful, global characteristics of the expression. These cells appear to respond to several attributes characteristic of the same expression. Similar expression-specific responses have also been described in the lateral nucleus of the amygdala.

Of all the facial features studied, it has been found that monkeys and humans are particularly sensitive to eye movements and the direction of gaze. Where another individual is looking is a good indicator of what he is thinking about: Such information can help us predict what he will likely do next. To test for responses to gaze direction, stimuli consisting of the faces of experimenters, doll faces, and slides of human and monkey faces were presented to monkey subjects from behind a shutter, at varying angles of head position and with varying angles of gaze direction. Researchers found that there were neurons responsive to specific angles of gaze in other monkeys or humans. Cells that were sensitive to direction of gaze were also sensitive to the direction in which the head was turned: The preferred direction of gaze was generally compatible with the preferred head direction. In other words, if a cell fired maximally in response to a set of eyes looking to the left, it also responded maximally to a head that was turned to the left.[14]

The identity of other individuals, their expression, and the direction in which they are looking provide meaningful social information to which brains must respond. What of body motion? What is interesting is that neurons code for motions of animate objects, such as the direction of head rotation, or the direction of a body motion—but these neurons are not sensitive to the motions of an *inanimate* object, such as large boxes or bars.[15] The neurophysiologist David Perrett showed that some of these cells were sensitive not only to the movement of a body through space, but could also use information derived from the movement of joints to derive the direction of a motion. I have studied how neurons respond to interactions between animals, by showing short movies of monkeys in natural settings, and it appears neurons respond to scenes in which monkeys approach or touch one another.[16]

Putting all these descriptions together is critical. A monkey or a human who had separate brain descriptions of "who" and "doing what" would be unable to respond quickly and correctly to the social situations in which it found itself. We know from anatomists' studies that separate pathways bearing motion and object information converge in the most forward part of the superior temporal sulcus.[17] Such information is likely to be relayed to temporal regions, such as entorhinal and perirhinal cortices, areas of the temporal lobe cortex that fold in and under the brain, wrapping around the amygdala and its neighbor the hippocampus. In these temporal regions, cells that responded to identity were found side-by-side with cells responsive to aspects of motion. One cell even responded both to identity and to the direction of head turns. It fired very quickly in response to moving pictures of a particular human individual, less quickly to pictures of a second individual, and not at all to other individuals, showing its ability to discriminate identity. But it also varied its firing rate depending on whether the pictured individuals were turning their heads toward, or away from, the viewing animal subject. And the difference in firing for the two directions was greater for one of the people than for the others.[18] The cell must have been receiving and integrating information both from identity-sensitive cells and from cells sensitive to the sight of bodily motion.

This region of the brain—the cortex that wraps around the front of the temporal lobe—is implicated in the laying down of memories, through connections with the hippocampal formation. Through its direct connections to other brain areas, it is also able to dictate bodily responses like hormone production and the cardiac and circulatory changes that accompany "fight or flight" reactions. The discovery of cells responsive to social features here suggests that, in primates, social events are doubly privileged. Registering them provides immediate access to storage in memory on the one hand, and immediate access to behavioral dispositions on the other.

From Laboratories to Jungles and Back

Because there are highly specialized neurons sensitive to such things as facial features and the direction of moving bodies, are there large systems of neurons specialized in these functions? We know that single neurons are components of large, distributed neural ensembles, whose overall patterns of activity encode both external stimuli and the animal's responses to them. The firing of a single neuron may reflect the activity of an entire ensemble from which it receives information. It may in addition belong to an ensemble whose overall activity specifies a feature of the environment in more detail than that neuron's activity alone. Thus, when the scientist's recording electrode encounters a selectively responsive neuron, he or she knows neural ensembles with at least the same degree of selectivity must also be active. The existence of *socially* specialized single neurons indicates that primates have entire neural ensembles that are specialized for registering social features of the environment. If this is so, would damage to, or removal of, brain tissue containing these ensembles produce specific disturbances of social behavior? Would artificial stimulation of these ensembles produce forms of social behavior?

The answer to both of these questions is yes, and the results reveal a highly developed social brain. But it was only when researchers studied the primate brain in a *social* context that they found its evolved, specialized functions—features that remained hidden as long as only the brains of isolated animals were studied.

The history of this work on the social brain began with just such isolated animals, however. In the 1930's, Heinrich Klüver and Paul Bucy made experimental lesions in the brains of singly caged laboratory monkeys to study vision. Like the visual neurophysiologists who stumbled across face-responsive cells some four decades later, they found themselves confronting unexpected and colorful results. The Klüver–Bucy syndrome is a set of behaviors seen in monkeys after surgical destruction of the anterior temporal lobes. In this syndrome, the caged animals become unusually tame, may place nonfood objects, including feces, in their mouths indiscriminately, and display unusual sexual behavior including mounting animals of other species. These behaviors can be produced by damage restricted to the amygdala alone, which suggests that the amygdala may be crucial, and the surrounding area less important, for producing the syndrome.

A neuroscientist, John Downer, demonstrated this in a dramatic way. He made a lesion in the amygdala (an "amygdalectomy") only on one side of a monkey's brain, and separated the two hemispheres of the brain surgically at the same time. As a result, the incoming visual information from each eye had access only to the hemisphere on the same side, and not to both, as is normally the case because of the visual system's crossing pathways. By closing first one of the monkey's eyes, and then the other, Downer showed that when the monkey saw the world with the eye connected to the intact side of the brain, he behaved in his usual aggressive manner toward humans. When the animal viewed the world only through the eye connected with the damaged amygdala, he was strikingly tame and docile. Downer's experiment demonstrated that the amygdala mediates the significance of visual input. Klüver and Bucy's results, together with Downer's, were taken to mean that the amygdala is essential for attaching appropriate emotional significance to environmental stimuli.[19]

But the significance of changes in the natural, social behavior of amygdalectomized animals did not receive much attention. Changes in sexual behavior and aggressiveness were initially interpreted simply as instances of a more general failure to attach emotional meaning to environmental stimuli. Lesion studies of the amygdala and anterior temporal lobes tended to focus on their roles in nonsocial tasks. It took a scientist with a new point of view to bring about a reevaluation of the amygdalectomy experiments, for it was not until the lesioned animals were studied in natural social settings, rather than in isolated cages, that the importance of their social difficulties was appreciated. The scientist responsible for this crucial reinterpretation of the Klüver-Bucy experiments has also pioneered the study of the social dimensions of the brain more generally.

In the early 1950s, a young draftee named Arthur Kling was stationed at the Walter Reed Army Graduate School of Medicine as a caretaker of laboratory animals. Because of his background in zoology, he was invited to carry out experiments with Leon Schreiner, who had set out to study the neural basis of aggression. Together they were able to show that amygdalectomy in cats produced docility. An Army film dated 1952 documents the surgical procedure of amygdalectomy, and its behavioral results in several species—namely, rhesus monkeys, cats, and agoutis (a large South American rodent).[20] One scene shows a group consisting of a cat, a monkey, and an agouti, all with lesions of the amygdala, sitting quietly together. The narrator states, "It is unlikely that these animals could survive in their natural environments." Indeed, these animals are not able to respond appropriately to a situation—specifically, contact with their natural enemies—which would be threatening to a normal animal.

Following medical training and specialization in psychiatry, Kling took a position at the Michael Reese Hospital in Chicago. There, in the

1960s, he obtained and began to work with the stumptail macaque, a monkey whose interactions with humans were dramatically different from those of the "standard" laboratory primate, the rhesus macaque. The relative docility of the stumptail toward humans made Kling realize that the rhesus monkey was not *the* paradigm of primate behavior. He began to appreciate the diversity of brains and behavior among the various species of primates, realizing the rhesus monkey was not a model for all of primate brain–behavior relations.[21] This led Kling to conduct comparative studies of the effects of brain lesions on the behavior of several primates in addition to rhesus monkeys, including stumptail macaques and vervet monkeys.

Instead of concentrating on a single species and refining his understanding of brain mechanisms with only that species, Kling used the plurality of results yielded by different species with their different brains and repertoires of behavior. Furthermore, he became interested in how lesions affected behavior at different stages of development, and in how the different contexts in which an animal was placed would affect the impact of a particular brain lesion on behavior. Throughout the next decade, the proposal made in the 1952 film remained in the back of his mind—namely, how would an animal with an amygdalectomy behave in its natural social environment?

Fortunately, resources were available to allow him to pursue this question. Having studied lesioned vervet monkeys in the lab, he sought an opportunity to extend his observations to the field. With funds from the Rockefeller Foundation, Kling set out to Zambia in 1968, to join Sherwood Washburn's student Jane Lancaster in her camp at Livingstone. In the meantime, he had also contacted Ronald Myers, then director of a National Institutes of Health research colony of rhesus monkeys in Puerto Rico. Between 1966 and 1971, a series of experiments were carried out in Puerto Rico to study the effects of lesions of various temporal lobe structures. What researchers found was that inferior and superior temporal lesions—areas of temporal cortex dedicated to visual and auditory perception, respectively—did not produce alterations in social behavior, so long as brain structures such as the amygdala and the cortex at the frontmost end of the temporal lobe, known as the temporal pole, were spared. In Zambia, Lancaster and Kling made surgical lesions of the amygdalas of vervet monkeys, then studied their behavior after returning them to their social groups in the wild. As controls they studied vervets that had been held in captivity for the same duration and then returned to the wild. The surgeries were carried out in a makeshift operating room set up in the kitchen of Lancaster's house in Livingstone.

What Kling and his colleagues learned was fascinating. Other vervets made friendly approaches to the operated-on vervets, even though they withdrew; in contrast, rhesus monkeys that had been operated on were commonly attacked, chased, and killed by other members of the group. Both rhesus and vervet monkeys, when lesioned, became socially isolated, however. The most significant result, though, was the total absence of the Klüver–Bucy syndrome in the wild in either rhesus or vervet monkeys, although both species showed this syndrome when isolated and caged. When operated animals were returned to the wild, they never attempted to place inappropriate material in their mouths. Hypersexuality was never seen, in contrast to the case of the caged animals. And rather than displaying the unusual tameness typical of caged lesioned animals, the released animals were inappropriately fearful, withdrawing from all friendly approaches by other members of the group to which they formerly belonged, eventually becoming completely isolated. Animals that had also been taken from the groups, but that were anesthetized without actually undergoing surgery, resumed their normal social behavior when reintroduced to the group in the wild. Thus it was clear that the socially withdrawn behavior resulted from lesions to the amygdala, and not just from the fact that the animals had been captured for a time. The point is that the classical Klüver–Bucy syndrome simply did not appear in lesioned monkeys in the wild.

This striking difference in the lesion's effect as a function of the social context in which the animals were studied highlights the importance of the social environment in mediating the effects of brain lesions. For one thing, the brains of monkeys that are experimentally isolated differ in their chemical makeup from those of monkeys housed in groups.[22] For another, monkeys have not been prepared by evolution for the kind of sensory stimulation they receive in isolated cages. Lesioned or intact, brains that evolved to carry out social interactions are not likely to be well understood when they are studied in the artificially isolated environment of the solitary cage. The Robinson Crusoe metaphor had impeded progress in understanding the primate brain; Kling's attention to the importance of sociality restored the brain to its proper context.

A variety of follow-up studies carried out in the 1970s by Kling and his colleagues, in both natural and captive settings, further documented the results of amygdala lesions. The effects of the lesions varied depending on the species and age of the subject: Juveniles, for example, often recovered social function as they matured. Fall in dominance rank and deterioration of maternal behavior were the rule; alterations in sexual behavior and affiliative behaviors such as grooming were also common. In sum, the behavior of lesioned primates depends on a number of factors, including the structure that is lesioned, the species, and the developmental stage of the animal. Most important, Kling proved how necessary it is to take into account whether the behavioral context in which an animal is studied is social or asocial.

Why is the amygdala so crucial for social behavior? A clue lies in the patterns of its connections to the rest of the brain. Because of neurons that project to it from other areas, it receives highly processed sensory information. In turn, its own neurons send signals to regions that produce bodily changes, such as altered heart rate and blood flow. Thus, it is a kind of interface between impressions coming in from outside and bodily states. It is well situated to produce rapid, finely tuned physical responses to external events—and *social* events may be the most critical and demanding external challenges monkeys confront, day in and day out.

But the amygdala is not alone in this pattern of connections to the rest of the brain. The orbital frontal cortex is similar in its pattern of inputs and outputs. Interestingly, the primatologist Michael Raleigh found that lesions of orbital frontal cortex also cause altered social behavior. He found that vervet monkeys with orbital frontal lesions decrease their social contact with one another. In addition, they change their previous social roles: For example, orbital-frontal-lesioned females reject juveniles, which is not their usual behavior. Lesions of orbital frontal cortex in rhesus monkeys produce aversion to social contact and a decrease in aggression. Thus, the amygdala and orbital frontal cortex, which are themselves interconnected, may be considered components of a social brain system. Based on observations from a number of researchers, Kling and his primatologist colleague H. Dieter Steklis proposed a neural system comprising the posterior orbital frontal cortex, the cortex of the temporal pole, and the amygdala as the basis of social bonding in monkeys.[23]

What if the amygdala and other brain regions that make up a specialized social system are stimulated? As we might expect, when electrical stimulation is experimentally applied to the amygdala, the cortex of the temporal pole, or the anterior cingulate gyrus, fragments of social behavioral routines result.

To stimulate small regions of the brain, electrodes are lowered into regions that investigators wish to study. Small amounts of current are passed through the tip of the electrode, below the level, which would destroy brain tissue, so that electrical activity is produced. Electrical stimulation can produce one of two effects. It can disrupt the orderly patterns of neural activity carried out by that region, in the same way that an electrical storm may disrupt normal patterns of electricity in a city. For example, human patients may become unable to speak during neurosurgery if the areas controlling speech are stimulated electrically. Alternatively, when applied in primary motor or sensory regions, electrical stimulation may mimic the effects of neural activity and produce movements or sensations. Many early discoveries of the functional organization of the brain began when it was discovered, for example, that stimulation of what is now known as the motor cortex produced body movements.[24]

In monkeys, stimulating social brain structures produces social behavior. If the anterior temporal region is electrically stimulated, a rhesus monkey will vocalize or make facial movements. Vocalizations also result from stimulating the amygdala of rhesus and other monkey species, or from stimulating the anterior cingulate gyrus. Penile erection may occur in response to amygdala stimulation, as well as components of fearful and defensive behavior, such as dilation of the pupils and raising of the hair. Thus the amygdala and its system appear to have a special role to play in complex social behavior—whether it involves sexuality, communication, or defense.[25]

Orderly sequences of facial displays, body postures, and vocalizations, when they appear in a specific social context, are meaningful messages from a monkey that signal to other monkeys what its intentions are. The ability both to understand those sequences and to emit them appropriately are essential to social survival in primates. Brain stimulation in the isolated laboratory situation produces only components of normal behavioral sequences. Vocalizations (such as calls and grunts), penile erections, and facial grimaces produced by brain stimulation are fragments of social response routines that, under natural conditions, would be evoked and strung together in appropriate sequences during social interactions. Although the simple application of electrical current cannot generate orchestrated sequences of complex behavior in isolated monkeys, it can produce orchestrated sequences if the stimulation is carried out in a social setting, as we will see in chapter 5.

In summary, we have seen that neurophysiological research, initially oriented to the brain as it functions in isolation, produced results that pointed unequivocally to the way it functions in social environments. Kling's research, which was focused on the importance of the social environment from the beginning, delineated which brain regions might be essential for primate social behavior. Together, these two lines of experimental work paved the way for a new perspective on the primate brain. The results we have surveyed so far pertain to the brains of various species of monkeys. It is time to take up the human social brain, and to look in more detail at its evolutionary history.

4

The Editor Speaks

What Patients Told their Doctors

Upon stimulating his left amygdala at 1mA, he had a feeling "as if I were
not belonging here," which he likened to being at a party and not being
welcome.

Right hippocampal stimulation at 3mA induced anxiety and guilt,
". . . like you are demanding to hand in a report that was due 2 weeks
ago . . . as if I were guilty of some form of tardiness."[1]

These sensations are those of a 20-year-old man who was undergoing
brain electrical stimulation while recounting his experiences out loud
to Dr. Pierre Gloor, a neurologist at the Montreal Neurological Institute. Like other patients whose epilepsy is unfortunately not able to be
controlled by medication, the young man had chosen to undergo
surgery to remove the part of his brain that was triggering the seizures.
To prepare for the surgery, his neurosurgeon had implanted electrodes
into the regions thought to be causing the seizures. These regions were
in the temporal lobes. The patient's brain activity was being recorded
directly from the electrodes over a period of time in the hospital and
correlated with the onset of his seizures, which were carefully moni-
tored. The correlations would guide the surgeon in the subsequent removal of the part of the brain causing the epilepsy. During this
diagnostic phase in the treatment of such patients, Gloor often ran
very small amounts of current into individual electrodes, to see
whether a patient's typical seizure symptoms were produced. If the
symptoms marking the onset of a patient's typical seizures were reproduced by electrical stimulation, then the site of stimulation would
probably also be the site of seizure onset—additional information that
is useful for the surgeon. Because Gloor's patients were alert and could

report their experiences, such stimulation procedures provided a unique opportunity to study the functions of the regions being stimulated—an opportunity he used to develop new insights. The verbatim accounts of this 20-year-old man are part of Gloor's invaluable contributions to our understanding of the social brain.

The context for understanding Gloor's contribution dates back to the 1950s. The neurologist Wilder Penfield and others had shown that stimulating a patient's temporal lobe cortex can cause perceptual experiences. These might be visual hallucinations such as seeing a face or a scene, auditory hallucinations such as hearing a voice or music, or hallucinations involving other senses such as bodily sensations, taste, or smell. Often the bodily sensations related to regions such as the chest or stomach and consisted of tightness or nausea. Subjective experiences such as fear had also been frequently evoked, especially when stimulating deeper temporal structures such as the amygdala. Bodily changes and intense subjective experiences might coincide, for example, a patient undergoing stimulation might turn pale, look fearful, and cry out. And even more striking observations had been made: Patients sometimes experienced brief, autobiographical memories involving familiar scenes. During these experiences, the patient had a sense of reliving something familiar.[2] As Gloor was to emphasize in his own writing, the remembered scenes did not unfold as stories, but were static in time. As an example of an evoked memory, the 20-year-old patient described above, when tested on another occasion, reexperienced a frightening event from his childhood: it took place in a park in Ottawa and involved being pushed into water by a bigger boy. During such experiences, which may also occur during spontaneous seizures, patients feel "as if they were there again." Thus it was known that stimulation of the temporal lobes could produce bodily changes, feeling states, and complex sensory impressions, separately or in combination.

Based on careful analysis of his own extensive stimulation studies, Gloor concluded that stimulation of the amygdala may not only give rise to all the above experiences, but that it does so more reliably than any other temporal lobe structure. But his new and profound insight related to the nature of the experiences themselves: he realized that the episodes are

> most often set in what might be called a "social context" in the broadest sense of the term, or better perhaps in an "ethological context." . . . They frequently bear some relationship with familiar situations or situations with an affective meaning. They frequently touch on some aspect of (the patient's) relationship with other people, either known specifically to him or not.[3]

In other words, experiences that have to do with *social interaction* can be generated in human patients by stimulating regions of the temporal lobes. And as the patient's words revealed, the reported experiences involve *feelings appropriate to certain social situations*—in the first the feeling of being an unwelcome stranger, and in the second the feeling of being found remiss by a superior. Such situations involve the actions, attitudes, or intentions of others, directed at oneself.

We can imagine how such social representations are created by the brain in actual experience, as opposed to the setting of electrical stimulation. In real-life experience, the sensory representations of the "others" are specific and spelled out, because external stimuli activate widespread areas of sensory cortex. For example, being at a gathering where you are unwelcome or where you do not know anyone would cause activation of widespread cortical representations of lights, sounds, faces, facial expressions, directions of gaze, and so on. These cortical ensembles converge in structures such as the amygdala, to activate appropriate patterns of neural activity. The bodily changes brought about by the resulting amygdala activity might include sensations of tightness in the chest or stomach, perspiration, and an increased heart rate. The combination of external sensory perception (the unexpressive gazes of strangers) with a bodily state (nervousness) represents a specific social situation *that includes as an aspect of it* an urgent disposition to act in some way (leave; find a familiar face; solicit a friendly gesture from someone). Furthermore, once the amygdala sets certain patterns into motion, these may feed back to the sensory cortex to create a bias on the information being received.[4] In the current example, once the sense of being ostracized is set in motion, benign social gestures may be perceived as unfriendly, that is, one feels "paranoid."

In the setting of the electrical stimulation, in contrast, only partial activation of social ensembles could occur, because of the absence of an objective external set of stimuli to activate sensory cortex. Thus, the patients do not experience full-fledged hallucinations, replete with sensory detail. Instead, they have "feelings."

There are two important points to be made regarding the patients' feelings. One is that the feelings are response dispositions—that is, tendencies to act—specifically tuned to particular social situations. Such tendencies might be fleeting and weak; or they might be fully coordinated, overt actions. Response dispositions arise by virtue of the connectivity of brain regions such as the amygdala and orbital frontal cortex to motor, endocrine, and autonomic brain regions, regions that set a blueprint for bodily states. The philosopher Daniel Dennett uses the example of uneasiness, which some individuals experience when seeing a snake, pointing out that this emotion is simply equivalent to "innate biases built into our nervous systems. These favor the release of adrenaline, bring fight-or-flight routines on line, and, by activating various associative links, call a host of scenarios into play involving danger, violence, damage."[5] Although our everyday use of terms such as "feelings" and "emotion" may seem to imply that they have a special essence—an existence over and above bodily states—there is no reason to think that anything other than dispositions to act are involved when we speak of feeling. Of course, not all feelings arise because of evolved predispositions. Associative links could also be created by one's personal life experience, giving rise to idiosyncratic reactive dispositions. Nevertheless, these too amount in the end to bodily states, preparations for response.

The second point is well illustrated by this patient. He resorted to describing social situations in order to convey his feelings to Gloor— for the simple reason that he had feelings he could not name. He relied on the neurologist being able to identify a feeling by *invoking a social situation in Gloor's imagination*. And it is a good strategy, for anyone reading or hearing the description of the situation understands: "Oh, *that* feeling." The strategy is also used by people who must explain certain feelings to foreigners: Requested to explain the meaning of a word for an attitude, a Pacific islander told the anthropologist, "That is the feeling one has when one has to stand up before others in meetings and speak."[6] From this description, we automatically identify the feeling, which we label stage fright or self-consciousness. The cross-cultural success of the strategy indicates that certain social feelings (and the social situations that induce them) belong to a common, evolved inheritance. These feelings are evolutionary products of the complex action situations that form the fabric of life in primate societies. They encode the appropriate responses to social situations, such as "stay with your own group, where you are known and will be responded to"; or "be submissive to the dominant individual who is upset with you"; or "avoid situations where many others are staring at you." The point is that our brains are evolutionarily prepared to generate certain responses to particular social situations. These responses are encoded in links between sensory representations of social events, and bodily changes—links that are found especially in the amygdala, where stimulation may produce feelings that are specifically appropriate for social situations.

Although systems for naming emotions vary greatly among different cultures, social feelings are not purely constructs of particular forms of thought. Indeed, some anthropologists, in agreement with the present position, have argued that there are innate emotional experiences lacking culturally prepared avenues for expression.[7] Social feelings are probably biologically based response tendencies that become elaborated and articulable through mediating concepts available in the family system and culture in which they occur. In the case of Gloor's patient, we must assume that his feelings were not independent of his own individual history. We do not know how much evolved, innate dispositions for perceiving certain social situations interact with individual learning to produce any given social response. But cross-cultural recognition of social situations, despite differences in labeling systems among cultures, suggests a common, evolved sensitivity to certain situations. I suspect Gloor's patient was not speaking metaphorically when he referred to being an uninvited guest, but was struggling to label a feeling for which he had no name.

If the anatomy of social responsiveness indeed involves neural ensembles that link highly processed sensory inputs with patterns of bodily activity, such as movements, hormone release, and fight-or-flight responses, then we would predict the following: Brain structures that have connections linking sensory cortices on the one hand, and motor, endocrine, and autonomic activity on the other, must be intact in order for adept, well-orchestrated social behavior to occur. The prediction holds true, as damage to brain regions with just this pattern of connectivity—historically termed "limbic" regions—causes specific social deficits. Our knowledge of the association between damage to limbic structures and social deficits is due in large part to the sophisticated use of brain-imaging technologies in combination with tests of cognitive function, as carried out by Antonio Damasio, Hanna Damasio, and their colleagues at the University of Iowa. Let's survey some of their findings regarding the effects of amygdala, orbital frontal, and cingulate damage on social behavior.

Natural lesions confined to the amygdala alone are extremely rare in humans. In most cases where the amygdala has been selectively destroyed by surgery, either little detailed comparison of preoperative and postoperative function is available, or the brain was clearly abnormal in unknown ways prior to surgery, making the results of surgery hard to assess. Detailed assessments of one nonsurgical patient with a rare disease causing damage to the amygdala alone were carried out by Damasio's colleagues Daniel Tranel and Bradley Hyman. They noted that the patient had a "tendency to be somewhat coquettish and disinhibited . . . and often makes mildly inappropriate sexual remarks."[8] Although this behavior suggests the role of the intact amygdala in social functioning, more specific social deficits were described in this patient as well. For example, she had difficulty recognizing expressions of fear in others, and blends of other facial expressions, although she was still able to recognize the identity of the faces.

A second patient with damage in the region of the amygdala also had difficulty deciphering facial expressions. This patient was tested to see if she could detect whether the eyes of a photographed face were looking directly at her, or slightly away. Compared to control subjects who were the same age, she had difficulty perceiving the direction of gaze.[9] The results from these two cases are consistent with the social impairments shown by monkeys with amygdala lesions. Researchers are beginning to test additional patients with amygdala damage, to see whether they too have difficulty reading social signals of various kinds.

For some time, neurologists have known that patients with orbital frontal lesions become inappropriately jocular without feeling real pleasure. They also are socially disinhibited—that is, they do not observe the normal conventions of behavior in public settings. The Iowa researchers characterized the deficits of such patients and a syndrome they called "acquired sociopathy" as exemplified by patient EVR. Prior to surgery for an orbitofrontal meningioma (a type of tumor) at age 35, the patient was an exemplary father, businessman, and member of his community. After the surgery, the patient retained a high level of intelligence, documented on numerous diagnostic tests, but became completely unable to make appropriate decisions regarding work, relationships, and daily living. He had a striking inability to assess the trustworthiness of new associates, and entered into partnerships with persons of doubtful character, resulting in his own bankruptcy. Further study revealed that EVR was able to solve difficult social problems, including sophisticated ethical problems, but only when presented with these verbally, and not in his actual life.

Finally, these researchers described a patient whose anterior cingulate region was damaged as a result of a stroke. In chapter 3 we saw that electrically stimulating the cingulate region in monkeys causes them to vocalize. Consistent with an evolved commonality in the social function of this area, human patients who have sustained damage to the cingulate become mute. Damasio's patient was able to talk about her experience after recovering, and said that she had been mute because nothing seemed to matter—she had "nothing to say."[10]

In sum, human patients with damage to the cingulate gyrus, amygdala, and the orbital frontal cortex are impaired in various ways in their social behavior. To be more specific about the anatomy of social cognition, however, we need to know how sensory representations of a social nature are encoded in cortical areas, for it is these representations that must be linked with response dispositions. Our information on the encoding of a very important category of social feature, facial expression, comes from an intriguing experiment in which neurosurgeons stimulated visual areas in the brain's right hemisphere.

In a study of visuospatial functions of the right hemisphere conducted by Itzhak Fried, George Ojemann, and their colleagues, visual memory tasks were given to eight patients whose brains were exposed under local anesthesia in preparation for subsequent surgery. As background for understanding their technique, it is necessary to know that neurosurgeons can "map" the functions various cortical brain regions serve by asking patients to perform certain language, visual, or memory tasks while the brain is being stimulated in the operating room. If the ability to do that specific task, but not others, is disrupted by localized cortical stimulation, then presumably the area being stimulated contributes in some crucial way to performing the task. Such studies are sometimes needed in cases where subsequent brain surgery is required, because the exact location of certain brain functions often varies from one individual to the next, and it is important to know exactly where speech, for example, is represented in a particular patient's brain, in order to avoid damaging that tissue. Such studies are rare, however, both because they can only be performed when clinically indicated, and because they are very difficult technically.

Social stimuli have seldom been used in studies such as these. As distractors during the memory tests, however, Fried showed the patients pictures of faces with emotional facial expressions numerous times. The patients were asked to choose a verbal label for the expression from the following list: neutral, happy, sad, anger, disgust, fear, and surprise. In the absence of electrical stimulation, patients made few errors in labeling the expressions. But with stimulation, particularly at sites in a localized region of the temporal cortex, they tended to name the expressions incorrectly. The errors revealed no consistent tendency to perceive expressions either more positively or negatively; furthermore, the ability to match pictures of the same faces, without respect to expression, remained intact. Thus, the deficit probably reflected neither a change in the attitude the patient was bringing to the task nor an error of facial perception per se, but rather, a deficit in the specific ability to perceive emotional expression. But the perception of oriented lines and neutral faces was impaired by stimulation in adjacent temporal regions, as was memory for those two categories of stimulus. Thus, the ability to perceive emotional facial expressions was shown to be localized to one region within the right hemisphere, with other visuospatial perceptual abilities being separately localized.[11]

Can we now offer an account of how the primate brain handles social cognition? Undoubtedly, distributed groups of neurons, whose stable firing patterns encode features of the outside world, extend from areas of the cortex supporting the early stages of sensory registration, to so-called "association" areas, where many aspects of a feature are combined in particular ways. Visual association areas tend in the case of object-related vision to be located toward the front end of the temporal lobe, and away from the occipital lobe in the back of the brain. The perception of a facial expression is more complex than the perception of a light–dark boundary: It depends on lower level visual processing (because damage to posterior visual areas causes blindness), but it must also depend on neural firing combinations that are formed at intermediate levels of visual processing—that is, in those parts of the neural ensemble that are found in the temporal lobes. Moreover, the ensembles that encode facial expressions are clearly in some ways separate from those that encode other complex visual patterns, as Fried's results demonstrated. This separateness is evidence for a specialization within the brain itself, a subsystem dedicated to *social* processing. I have used the term "editor" as a shorthand for this specialization. It is time to make the term more explicit.

The Nature of the Editor

We have seen in these first three chapters that researchers and clinicians working with humans and nonhuman primates pondered over results from single neurons, lesions, innate disorders, and electrical stimulation—all of which speak to a specialized capacity for social processing. What we need to make the picture complete is an account of the editor's mechanism. How did it evolve and how does it work?

The brain's social editor is an anatomical system consisting of the amygdala (and, to a lesser degree, related structures such as the orbital frontal cortex, anterior cingulate gyrus, and temporal pole cortex) and the sensory cortex reciprocally connected with it. As we know by this point, the amygdala is a cluster of neuron groups situated at the front end of the temporal lobes in both hemispheres. The anatomic relationship between the amygdala and the brain areas responsible for sensory information has only recently come to be fully appreciated. Generalizing from the fact that the rodent amygdala receives prodigious amounts of information from the olfactory bulb, it was originally believed that the amygdala's functions are primarily olfactory—having to do with smell. Primates and other mammals are believed to have descended from insectivores (insect eaters), present-day examples of which are creatures such as shrews, moles, and hedgehogs. The amygdala of insectivores indeed played an important role in integrating olfactory information, which is critical for both food location and social communication in such animals. The importance of olfaction in social communication is apparent today in some species of primates that are dependent on their sense of smell for several important functions as in some lemurs, for example, that communicate by scent-marking. Because the amygdala processes olfactory information in animals that use olfaction for social communication, it is obvious that it would have a special role in social communication in those animals.

Like their precursors the insectivores, early primates were mostly nocturnal. For mutual social regulation in insectivores and primitive nocturnal primates, the amygdala and its connections with olfaction were available. But as primates gradually became more dependent on vision, nature acted opportunistically, taking in hand available brain structures and tweaking them in new directions. Shedding their nocturnal habits, primates developed into highly social creatures, using their faces and other visual displays to deliver streams of rapid, flexible signals. In step with this ecological shift, nature enhanced the amygdala's capabilities, downplaying its erstwhile olfactory interests and upgrading its connections to other senses, including vision, audition (hearing), and sensations such as touch. As the amygdala became more connected with visual and auditory areas, the arrangement of nerves and muscles in the primate face also changed, giving it the capacity for expressiveness (compare our smiles to those of the hedgehog!), and all the while primate social groups were becoming more complex. The transmitting equipment—expressive faces—and the receiving equipment—sensory brain wired to the amygdala—were evolving in step, prodded on by the demanding social milieu.

The changes that the primate brain has undergone have been carefully documented by the anatomist Heinz Stephan and his colleagues, who conducted comparative studies of individual brain structures such as the amygdala across many species of insectivores and primates. They have evaluated these structures in terms of their relative size (that is, taking body size into account) and in terms of their differentiation—the degree of organization and delineation of their neural architectures. Their results show that, from insectivores through prosimians and nonhuman simians to humans, there is a clear increase in the relative size of the amygdala. However, subregions of the amygdala associated with olfaction are smaller in primates—even in primates that use olfaction—than they are in the insectivores.

Where did the increase in total size of the amygdala, from insectivores to humans, come from, then? Stephan and his co-workers found
that the lateral part of the amygdala—that is, the part that receives input from sensory and association areas of the cortex—increased
greatly in size. Others had recorded the fact that the expansion of the
cortex seems to be the hallmark of brain evolution in humans, who
have about three times as much cortex in relation to body size as do
nonhuman primates. The increase occurs primarily in the association
areas and in the prefrontal cortex. Thus, the expansion of the lateral
amygdala in primates has occurred in step with the expansion of the
association cortex.[12]

Studies looking at brain anatomy confirm that the amygdala and association cortex share reciprocal connections. In particular, the lateral
nucleus of the amygdala receives input from advanced levels of sensory
processing in the case of vision, audition, and body sensations, but
only primitive and superficial inputs from the olfactory system. Other
parts of the amygdala send return projections to even more widespread areas of the cortex, reaching back into the earliest processing
areas. Connections within the amygdala itself form the final link in a
dynamic chain, a chain that may selectively highlight incoming sensory
information.[13]

How is incoming information highlighted? Recall that neurons
work collectively, as large ensembles, to encode aspects of the world.
When the memory of a particular episode is invoked, subsets of neurons that were active together during the episode are reactivated,
thereby recreating a representation of the event. The reactivation can
occur under the guidance of smaller sets of neurons that had links to
that particular ensemble, but not links to ensembles representing other
episodes. Areas of the brain implicated in memory—anterior temporal
lobe structures—that have widespread reciprocal connections to cortex may be thought of as the driver of a carriage who holds the reins
controlling representational horses, encouraging some, and checking
others. The amygdala's "reins" are its projections to cortex.

But the amygdala is itself part of a system. The lateral nucleus of the
amygdala projects not only to other nuclei in the amygdala, but also to
the entorhinal cortex, a waystation that gathers sensory information and
transmits it to the nearby hippocampus—a memory center that inte-
grates patterns of neural activity for later recall. The entorhinal cortex is
especially large and differentiated in humans compared to other primates.[14] By virtue of its inputs from amygdala and sensory cortices, its
two-way links to the hippocampus, and its widespread projections back
to cortex, the entorhinal region and its surrounding cortex, like the driver

with reins in hand, probably also plays a role in selecting particular neural ensembles in widely distributed cortical areas.[15] Thus, the amygdala, hippocampus, entorhinal cortex, and other areas such as orbital frontal cortex work together to organize, stabilize, and lay down for future recall distributed networks of neurons encoding relevant features of experience in the cortex. The fact that these linking structures have elaborated their interconnectedness with the cortex, shifting away from an exclusive preoccupation with olfactory information, shows how the primate brain has extended its machinery for the conduct of social regulation to include large regions of the sensory brain.

Brain structures such as the amygdala and entorhinal cortex do not simply register coincident activity in cortical regions, passively hooking groups of neurons together. I have asserted that the editor is *biased.* The system of which the amygdala is part does not just "read" from the cortical blackboard: Instead, it lets some marks fade, and highlights and circles others. How does this happen?

We know that the organization of sensory experience in our brains changes as a result of learning. The neuroscientist Michael Merzenich and his colleagues studied properties of the auditory cortex in owl monkeys trained to respond to certain tonal frequencies.[16] After training, the size of cortex devoted to mapping the target frequencies had increased. Furthermore, individual neurons were more sharply tuned to the target frequencies after training than they had been before training (that is, they were more specifically responsive to their "best" frequencies, compared to other frequencies). Monkeys that heard the same sounds passively, as opposed to those that had to pay attention in order to earn a reward, did not show changes in their cortical representations of the presented frequencies. Thus, attention appeared to be critical for bringing about changes in the characteristics of the neural assemblies encoding experience.

Using guinea pigs, the neuroscientist Norman Weinberger found that when certain tones were made significant for the animals, by pairing them with mild electrical shock, neurons in primary auditory cortex shifted their tuning from previously preferred tones to the frequency of the significant tones.[17] Just as in the owl monkey experiments, the sensory part of the guinea pig cortex increased its responsiveness to those specially significant tones, over others. (Although the experiment used a negative reinforcement—a shock—it is also possible that the significance of the tone could have been created by a positive unconditioned stimulus as well.)

Weinberger speculated that the amygdala participates in organizing the tuning of guinea pig auditory cortex, by becoming activated in response to the shock. At the same time that auditory signals are arriving in cortex, the amygdala relays its activity to a brain region (the nucleus basalis), which also sends projections widely to regions of cortex. The activity of the nucleus basalis, via its neurotransmitter acetylcholine, would enhance the patterns of firing that are just then taking place, strengthening them in preference to other patterns in auditory cortex. Thus, sensory signals (the tone) arrive via sensory pathways, while "amplifying" or "Remember this!" signals arrive from the nucleus basalis, in response to signals from the amygdala. Both converge on the same place, the auditory cortex. The idea that the nucleus basalis is involved receives support from experiments in which acetylcholine is manipulated directly. Applying acetylcholine to auditory cortex, or blocking acetylcholine receptors there, respectively enhances or blocks both neural responses to auditory stimulation, and receptive field changes.

What about vision? Does the amygdala provide a route that enhances attention to particular features of the visual environment? Experiments analogous to Weinberger's, but that use visual instead of acoustic stimuli, have not been done. We know, however, that the amygdala's neurons send connections directly to regions of visual cortex. It is likely, therefore, that the amygdala could act to engrave certain significant patterns into visual cortices just as Weinberger showed that it does in auditory cortices. It could do so indirectly, by activating the nucleus basalis, or directly, by the signals its own neurons relay back to visual areas.

As an example, suppose I meet someone and have a very unpleasant interaction with that person. During our encounter, the person's facial features are being registered in my visual cortices, in a widespread pattern of neural activity. At the same time, because of the nature of the interaction between us, linking regions in my brain—such as my amygdala—are active, preparing my body for fight or flight. My amygdala, in addition to sending signals that affect my bodily state, is also sending signals to the nucleus basalis. The nucleus basalis showers my sensory brain with acetylcholine (including the parts of my brain that register voices and motions), encouraging the patterns of activity now active to become stably linked. As a result, the particular neural pattern associated with this particular face and voice will become easy to reactivate as an overall pattern. The amygdala's own neural projections back to visual and auditory cortices during the interaction enhance the pattern as well. And the next time I am upset, perhaps for reasons entirely unrelated to my current unpleasant encounter, the activity of my amygdala may reignite the sensory patterns laid down at the time of the encounter. Weeks later, in my depressed or worried state, the face and voice of this individual may come to my mind to preoccupy me.

In the laboratory, it is possible to make an event significant for an animal by artificial means. In contrast, if I meet someone and we exchange angry words, an electric shock is not needed to make that event important to me. Most events that are significant to animals have been significant for long periods of the animal's evolutionary history; these events are significant because *perceiving them enhances the organism's chances of survival and reproduction.* Animals whose brains are set to attend preferentially to and represent these events increase their chances of surviving and reproducing. The laboratory experiments described here show us how the amygdala might organize the brain to register certain events, in a context in which those events have been made significant artificially. Left to its own devices in the natural world, it is probable that the amygdala uses similar mechanisms to organize cortical representation so as to register events preferentially that are evolutionarily significant—in the case of primates these would be social events. The example I used just now invoked a particularly unpleasant social experience. It is likely, however, that faces, voices, and social actions are significant *in themselves*, eliciting amygdala activation through evolutionarily inscribed pathways, activation that in turn writes the social experience of the moment into an enduring neural assembly. I used the experiments of Merzenich and Weinberger in auditory areas to show how the tuning of neural assemblies in visual areas of the brain, and thus, the nature of the complex stimuli to which many of them respond, might be set by the amygdala. The social editor, in sum, is a set of structures in the anterior temporal lobe and areas related to it that evolved to select certain neural ensembles in sensory cortices—ensembles that encode social features—and link them to action dispositions.

We return once more to autism. Imaging studies have shown that, in some autistic individuals, there are abnormalities in a region at the back of the brain called the cerebellar vermis and in the cerebral cortex. Researcher Eric Courchesne has proposed that abnormalities of the cerebellum lead to other abnormalities in other areas of the brain through the loss of connections during development. Microscopic studies of autistic brains have shown a decrease in the number of certain cell types in the cerebellum and an increased number of small densely packed cells in areas including the hippocampus, amygdala, and entorhinal cortex. During the first 6 months of life, neurons migrate within the developing brain to take up their proper position. It is theorized that, during this phase, orderly migration in the brain of the autistic infant is disrupted. It is likely that the neurons of the amygdala are affected, but it has not been shown that these are the sole abnormalities to be found in microscopic or imaging studies of the autistic brain.[18]

Yet an animal model with many autistic-like features was created by lesioning a region that includes both the amygdala and the neighboring hippocampal formation in infant monkeys. Consistent with the findings of previous lesion studies reviewed in chapter 3, the author of the study noted that juvenile monkeys with this brain lesion remained socially isolated and withdrew from other monkeys. More detailed observation revealed, in addition, that they had blank facial expressions, poor body language, and lack of eye contact, paralleling disturbances in autism. They had more temper tantrums when placed in novel situations than did controls, and showed locomotor stereotypes such as twirling in circles, behaviors that are frequently present in autism. Follow-up studies with more restricted lesions showed that damage specifically in the amygdala and surrounding cortex (entorhinal and perirhinal cortices) is critical for producing autistic-like behavior. These experiments strongly suggest that dysfunction occurring during infancy in the amygdala—or in an interconnected system of which the amygdala is a part—produces autistic behavior.[19] In normal infants, by contrast, the functioning editor causes attention to be paid to faces, which results in extensive representation of faces, their movements, and the sounds they make. These representations are building blocks for the subsequent understanding of person and mind.

Prozac and Other Mood-Altering Drugs: An Emerging Link among Mood, the Brain, and Social Behavior

Serotonin, a naturally occurring chemical that acts as a neurotransmitter in the brain, is of general interest because of its probable role in human psychiatric disorders. Medications known as serotonin reuptake inhibitors, which include fluoxetine hydrochloride (Prozac), sertraline hydrochloride (Zoloft) and paroxetine hydrochloride (Paxil), among others, are presumed to cause an increase of serotonin activity in the brain. It is anecdotally reported that these medications have positive effects not only on mood, but on sociality as well. How did researchers zero in on the links between serotonin, limbic brain structures, and social behavior?

In 1976 scientists found a relationship between low serotonin in cerebrospinal fluid and violent suicide attempts in psychiatric patients. These findings were extended and refined by further discoveries that, in humans, impulsive aggression and low central serotonin levels are positively correlated. A similar relationship between central serotonin and aggression has also been demonstrated in monkeys. A group of free-ranging male rhesus monkeys were rated both behaviorally for aggressiveness, and by counting the number of wounds and scars, which are usually the result of fights. Using these measures, the group of 28 monkeys was ranked for aggressiveness and for serotonin in their cerebrospinal fluid. The result was significant—aggressiveness was linked to low serotonin levels. Conversely, in a different study, high serotonin activity in cerebrospinal fluid was correlated with affiliative sociality. In vervet monkeys, socially successful males use aggression sparingly. Some vervet males, however, may choose inappropriate targets, such as juveniles, or may tend to prolong fights unnecessarily. Pharmacologic depletion of serotonin produces such inappropriate aggressive behavior in male vervet monkeys. Thus, in humans, rhesus monkeys, and vervet monkeys, there is a link between low serotonin levels and inappropriate aggression.[20]

Serotonin levels have also been correlated with the achievement of social dominance by male vervet monkeys. (Roughly speaking, the dominance rank of a monkey can be assessed by the degree to which other monkeys yield it access to preferred resting spots, food, or mates.) Longitudinal studies of vervet monkeys reveal that high male dominance is correlated with appropriate as opposed to inappropriate aggression and with effective prosocial behavior, including the formation of alliances with dominant females. In an important experiment, the male dominance hierarchy in a vervet monkey social group was rendered uncertain by removal of the dominant male. Males in the group who were treated with serotonin ultimately attained dominance. In a repeat experiment, when the same individuals were given serotonin-inhibiting drugs, they showed low-dominance behaviors instead. The sequence by which serotonin-treated males became dominant, through alliances and affiliative behavior, was identical to the sequence by which vervet males become dominant under natural conditions.[21]

The primatologists Michael Raleigh and Gary Brammer studied the individual behavioral styles of a group of adult male vervet monkeys by counting and classifying the interactions they had with other members of their group. Then they sacrificed the monkeys and searched their brains for a particular kind of serotonin receptor (a site on the surface of neurons where serotonin molecules attach, triggering the neurons to become active) known as the S-2 receptor. They found striking relationships between S-2 receptor numbers in the posterior orbital frontal cortex and the amygdala of individual brains, and stable patterns of affiliative and aggressive behavior they had previously observed in these monkeys. The number of S-2 receptors in the posterior orbital frontal cortex correlated strongly with measures of affiliation and were inversely correlated with rates of initiating or escalating aggression. The number of S-2 receptors in the amygdala was significantly linked to grooming (a behavior important in establishing affiliative relationships in monkeys), and nearly significantly linked to proximity, that is, the time an animal spends near others, and inversely tied to the tendency to escalate fights.[22]

The significance of these findings is that, for the first time, a possible anatomical basis for the social effects of serotonin has been found using systematic measures of primate behavior. The Raleigh and Brammer findings suggest how variations in the function of orbital frontal cortex and amygdala, resulting from different levels of serotonin, might affect primate social behavior. And it is likely, given the congruence between findings in humans and in monkeys relating serotonin levels and social behavior, that the serotonergic brain systems of vervet monkeys and humans function in similar ways.

The implications of the evolved social brain are not necessarily positive. Recall that the experiences evoked by stimulating the amygdala in human patients were mostly unpleasant ones—experiences of being intimidated, rejected, or criticized by others. This is consistent with animal studies, in which amygdala stimulation often produces aggressive and defensive routines. It is also consistent with anecdotal evidence that patients whose amygdalas are missing altogether (whether because of selective damage or more widespread damage to the temporal lobes) tend to be happier, and more carefree in their general attitudes. In other words, our brain's specialization for producing social responses seems to have a bias toward negative situations, as though evolution placed a premium on our ability to shrink in submission, bristle in retaliation, or retreat from others' indifference. Some of us may register these unpleasant feelings too frequently and in ways that are inappropriate to the circumstances—to our detriment. Thus we perceive others as critical, antagonistic, or rejecting. Correspondingly, our body states register fear, reactive irritability, or dejected withdrawal. Our brains are like hypervigilant sentries on duty in the dark, perceiving malevolence in every rustle of the bushes.

From observations of my own patients, I have come to think that increases in brain serotonin might act by dampening the activity of social brain structures. This in turn may cause a nonspecific suppression of bodily reactivity, impacting feeling states generally, including—in some cases—sexual function. Patients notice that the automatic negative social responses they previously experienced and expressed fade away. Those who benefit from serotonin-increasing medicines feel less anxious in social situations, less irritable, and less withdrawn. In some cases, they may notice a tendency to enjoy more prolonged social contact, such as casual conversation, or even a tendency to increased jocularity. It would be interesting to know whether these medicines can produce a full-fledged syndrome of complete insouciance resulting in poor social judgment, as seen in patients with orbital frontal and large temporal lesions described by Antonio Damasio. I have not personally seen this effect from serotonin-reuptake inhibitors. Instead, I have observed that increased serotonin in a previously troubled individual produces effects that parallel those seen in a colony of vervet monkeys—less pointless wrangling, more affiliative behavior, and improved relationships.

5

The Shift to a Social Perspective

Isolated Mind, Isolated Brain

Neuroscientists want to understand how the brain produces behavior. They ask how the brain makes it possible for us to perceive objects, to attend to and remember events, to reason. Like all scientists, their goal is to seek ever-more-accurate knowledge of the natural world—in this case, brain function—by formulating testable hypotheses and testing them in a way that can be reproduced and discussed by the scientific community. Underpinning this goal is the concept of a reality that is "out there," independent of us, that our minds may grasp and come to know, just as we use our eyes to grasp visually what is before us. The idea that there is a relationship between a mind and the things outside it in the world is the essence of the natural sciences—it is the faith in human knowledge. Although it was explicated most vigorously and confidently in the Enlightenment, contemporary empirical sciences are still grounded in the idea of this basic relationship.

But the idea not only determines the practices and procedures of neuroscience, it has also provided a metaphor for the brain itself. The brain has been implicitly seen as a "knower" of the world, as a socially isolated organ whose purpose is to grasp the inanimate world outside it. Modern systematic philosophy is rooted in the idea that our relationship to objects is analogous to visual perception.[1] Consistent with the conceptual power of the metaphor of brains as isolated Enlightenment minds is the considerable dominance of the study of vision in the neurosciences, which continues to this day.

The initial reluctance to place the brain in a social context was determined by other, practical, factors as well. Social environments consist of complicated beings that move about and signal to each other in complicated ways. Social stimuli, in common parlance, are "messy." They make trouble for well-designed experiments, which must simplify and control for everything that affects the animal or human under study. If during an experiment there are extraneous noises, or other persons or monkeys moving about, or even complicated rather than simple things to look at, it becomes hard to evaluate the subject's brain activity. The brain might be responding to something other than the situation the experimenter set out to test. This is the reason that the experimental situation must be carefully *controlled.*

Therefore, controlled experiments on higher brain function in nonhuman primates traditionally consisted of an isolated monkey faced with a series of challenges in the form of inanimate objects. For example, the animal was trained to fix its gaze on a spot on a screen before it while attending to a blinking line or circle in its peripheral visual field. As this visual or memory task was being carried out, brain activity was measured to test a hypothesis regarding the neural basis of visual perception or spatial memory. The reason for putting an animal in such an unnatural setting was to restrict the stimuli to which its brain was exposed. Using this sort of experimental environment created two problems, however; first, it assumed that a monkey's brain was the same whether the animal was isolated or in a social setting, an assumption we now know is incorrect.[2] Second, it asked only nonsocial questions about the animal's brain. This was like taking apart a watch to discover why it makes a ticking noise, but failing to appreciate how the gears function to keep time. The scope of the inquiry, in other words, limited scientists to only a certain kind of understanding.

Earlier we reviewed how biologists progressively came to understand the substance initially known as chromatin, which had been identified in the nuclei of cells, and how their understanding ultimately enabled them to unravel the mysteries of inheritance and differentiation. Imagine what would have happened if biologists studying inheritance had made a wrong assumption. Let us suppose that, because of some mistaken preconception, the chromatin they discovered was thought to be some confounding artifact, an interference with the "true" functions of the cell. Let us suppose biologists believed that, in order to understand cells, they must first rid them of this messy-looking material. Imagine that they were able to achieve this purification, and that, ever after, the model cell used for virtually all investigations was the chromatin-less cell. How far we would now be from understanding the material basis of genetic transmission!

We now know that the human brain, considered in isolation from its social functions, is like a cell without chromatin. One may learn many things by studying the DNA-less cell, but one will never learn how organisms arise from eggs and sperm. One may likewise learn many things about an isolated brain, but one will never learn how self, belief, and the communication that makes these and other things public are possible. By excluding from consideration the essential sociality of human beings, a purely artificial conundrum was perpetuated—for the human brain, stripped of its intrinsic sociality, is in fact mindless. This was the central paradox of mind/brain philosophy prior to the emergence of the social paradigm. It generated a great deal of mystification.

In chapter 3, I introduced Robinson Crusoe's reaction to the footprint as a literary version of the amazement experienced by visual scientists when they first discovered socially responsive cells. Robinson Crusoe is also a metaphor for the mystification the isolated brain concept produces. The fable presents him as essentially isolated, his existence dependent only on the manipulation of the nonhuman, natural world. But constructing Robinson Crusoe as an isolated mind depends on ignoring the history of socialization he brought with him to his exile. Similarly, considering an individual's behavior as the product of his or her isolated "mind" depends on ignoring the extensive socialization that produces organized thought and behavior in every human being, socialization for which our brains are innately prepared. It denies the fact that mind is a social creation to begin with, a creation made possible by our brains' adaptation for social participation.

The mystification produced by the isolated-mind fallacy was probably compounded by another mystification—the claim that science is purely progressive and acultural, and that scientists' ideas are free from social influences.[3] Scientists derive their status and legitimacy from such claims, and neuroscientists are no exception. It is possible that asociality was projected from neuroscience's collective self-image onto the brain. Because the brain as construed by neuroscience is held to be the organ of human nature, the threatened upshot of this projection was that human nature would be construed as asocial as well.

But if this idea had ever been stated explicitly, it would have been rejected of course. We grow up in families, interact with bosses and co-workers, have friends, meet strangers, and successfully carry out hundreds if not thousands of mini-interactions daily—besides the conversations and interactions we carry on inside our own heads with imagined others when we are alone. The requirement for sophisticated cognition in all this is immense. Nevertheless, the asocial view of the brain did not immediately strike everyone as nonsense. Why was this? It was probably because we carry out complex social maneuvers so easily, and they affect and permeate our feelings so completely, that we hardly notice them. In the same way that breathing through gills would be transparent to a fish, our sociality is all but transparent to us because it is continuous and part of how we are constituted. In sum, the fact that our sociality is so pervasive as to be taken for granted, together with the need for experimental control and a philosophical tradition of considering the mind to be asocial—all these contributed to scientists' initial reliance on an isolated-mind model in their investigations of the primate brain.

Scientists Take on a Challenge

In chapter 3, we saw that vision experiments yielded unexpected findings. Socially responsive neurons stepped onto the stage like characters from another play, speaking lines written by a different playwright. Unlike the well-behaved neurons carrying out low-level visual tasks, these interlopers seemed to be complex and specialized. Furthermore, the initial few lines that they spoke, and the additional things they were induced to say, hinted at a different kind of story, a story about primates' evolutionary history in a world of other primates. Like the footprint on Crusoe's island, the "hand cell" recorded in Gross's laboratory was the harbinger of a dramatic change from an isolated to a social view of the brain.

How did neuroscientists accommodate Gross's startling findings? It was difficult at first. Recall that his neurons, responsive to complex objects such as faces and hands, were believed to be compatible with a theory of encoding in which simple features of the environment combined in a hierarchical chain to produce so-called "grandmother cells," cells that could be triggered by specific, complex objects. We saw that this theory of encoding was abandoned by the scientific community a few years after Gross described the cells. Scientists currently believe simple features are represented in a distributed fashion across large numbers of neurons, and complex objects are represented only at the ensemble level. Because the principle of encoding at the level of the ensemble rather than the neuron became the predominant idea within a few years after Gross's "hand cell" and subsequent "face cells" were discovered, his findings became a challenge to received ideas. The triggers for these cells seemed too much like complex objects, and not enough like simple features.

Scientists were quick to raise the possibility that the brain might have a specialized system for face encoding, however. They drew a connection between face-responsive single neurons in monkeys and an interesting neurological syndrome affecting a small number of human

patients. The syndrome, called prosopagnosia, or more simply, face agnosia, results from brain injuries, often strokes, which damage certain
regions.[4] Patients with face agnosia vary in their deficits, depending on
the exact location of their injury. Generally, they remain relatively
unimpaired in most aspects of functioning, and have normal visual
abilities, but are unable to identify familiar faces. Thus, in tests using
photographs of known faces such as their own spouses or children, in-
termixed with unknown faces, these patients firmly state that none of
the faces are known to them. Often, the inability to recognize an individual is limited to problems in face recognition, because on hearing
the person's voice or even when watching their characteristic mode of
walking, these patients can immediately identify the familiar person.
Thus, when neurons that responded specifically to faces were discovered in monkeys, it was theorized that they belonged to a system that
was specialized to respond to faces, perhaps the same system that produced face agnosia when damaged in humans. Conversely, neurologists studying prosopagnosia cited studies of face cells in monkeys.

But science's path is never straight. As studies of face agnosia progressed, difficulties arose. It became clear that at least some patients
were impaired in their abilities to recognize nonface objects as well.
Recognition problems surfaced in cases in which there were many objects that were quite similar in configuration. For example, a woman
with prosopagnosia also could not recognize her own house. Thus,
face agnosia came increasingly to be studied as an impairment of recall
based on visual cues, not as a socially specific defect of visual perception. As it became clearer that prosopagnosia could affect nonface objects, the emphasis in the single-neuron literature also shifted away
from the notion of a specialized system for faces. Another reason for
the shift was that there was not a clear correspondence between the regions in which face-responsive cells were being found in monkeys, and
the regions in humans that, when damaged, caused face agnosia. Furthermore, when the "face cell" region in monkeys was removed, they
showed no difficulties discriminating between or identifying faces.[5]
They did have difficulty identifying gaze direction, however.

Scientific articles published over an interval of about 7 years revealed the course of scientists' struggles to come to grips with face
cells. Robert Desimone and his colleagues concluded a 1984 article by
noting that most neurons in inferotemporal cortex are not specifically
responsive to complex stimuli. Therefore, consistent with the theory of
distributed encoding, the encoding of visual objects occurs across a
population of inferotemporal neurons, in a particular pattern of activity,
and not in the activity of individual cells. They noted that cells selective

for faces were an apparent exception to this rule. In this article, they speculated that there has been selective pressure on primates giving rise to specialized neural systems for recognizing faces, and that deficits in such a system would also be the basis of prosopagnosia. In a review published in 1991, Desimone took into account the newer findings in prosopagnosia regarding difficulties with nonface objects. He considered that faces were only different from other objects in being so extensively experienced by monkeys. He, and likewise Gross, concluded that face-responsive cells, rather than being an exception, might actually be a model of the visual recognition of complex objects generally. The discovery of neurons in the brains of sheep that responded specifically to the sights of both sheep and dog faces, seemed to support the idea that a brain will develop specialized cells for any class of object that is seen frequently. According to this line of thinking, faces are simply a very common object and face perception can be used to understand how vision works in general.[6] The emphasis of Gross's and Desimone's research had originally been on mechanisms of vision. After a brief shift to the idea of a social specialization, the emphasis returned to vision once again.

But researchers could not ignore the emerging social framework. It is a basic tenet that brains cannot be understood apart from the environment in which they evolved. Humans, and before them their hominid ancestors, have always been born into and lived in social groups. Unlike some other animals, no human infant can survive without others of its kind to care for it. Newborns actively seek out faces with their gaze, showing that they are ready from birth to acquire vast experience with the human face—and later, as auditory and linguistic mechanisms mature, with the sounds that issue from it. In infancy and adulthood, humans have always had, and still have, extensive experience with the appearances and actions of other humans. In the ordinary, expectable environment of evolution, the human brain encodes social events, and encodes them extraordinarily well.

This means that during our species' history, through the usual evolutionary processes of mutation and selection, there arose neural mechanisms especially good at registering social features—faces, for example. Neural mechanisms do not "care" about the exact nature of the work they do, however. They process information at a more abstract level than the raw features of the stimuli themselves. So, just because our brains are extraordinarily adept at perceiving faces, it does not follow that the neural mechanisms involved would balk at performing nonface tasks that are analogous in their processing. By testing brain-damaged patients who can't perceive faces with analogous perceptual tasks, researchers have been able to demonstrate parallel deficits in the perception of other stimuli. Using such techniques, they are beginning to understand the abstract aspects of the processes that underlie face recognition. Therefore, in the sense that neural mechanisms are indifferent to the actual content of stimuli, faces are not "special" as far as the brain is concerned. But to the extent that primate sociality drove brains to develop these particular processes in the first place, and to the extent that our brains' highly developed social tuning produces many very significant consequences, faces are indeed special. [7]

Little by little, scientists began to acknowledge that the importance of faces is a condition of life for primates, that sociality is a very important context in which to study primates—not an accidental variable to be excluded, especially when the goal is to understand human thought. By accepting this new framework, they began to see that the *social* environment has produced an important specialization of brain function in human beings. I have likened this development to the rotation of the reptilian jaw bones that created a new perceptual organ, the mammalian ear. By generating the concepts of persons and selves, the social organ of the primate brain produces immensely significant effects. It makes all the difference in the world that our brains have a special sensitivity to the sights and sounds of our fellow beings, as opposed to the sights and sounds of some aspect of the inanimate world, such as leaves or rocks. For the social brain not only senses, it also *creates* social worlds.

The dialogue in the scientific literature over the face-recognition cells illustrates how science works. Unexpected findings strain existing paradigms. Back and forth struggles regarding the proper context and significance of the findings ensue. Ultimately—sometimes after many years of discussion—old frameworks for understanding are replaced by new ones. The replacement takes place not because the old ones were wrong, but because the new ones are more useful. Moreover, during such transitions it is not unusual to find new and old frameworks operating side by side. A social framework for understanding primate brains did not arise de novo with Gross's discoveries. Indeed, some years before he found socially selective neurons, when the isolated brain approach was in full ascendance, a few scientists had already intuitively begun to use social contexts to study the primate brain.

We saw in chapter 3, for example, that Arthur Kling pioneered the use of lesion studies in a social setting in the late 1960s. He showed that amygdala lesions affected the behavior of monkeys very differently when they were isolated and caged than when they were placed in social groups: The Klüver–Bucy syndrome is an artifact of isolation. We also saw in chapter 3 that bits of social behavior could be produced by electrically stimulating the brains of isolated, restrained monkeys in the laboratory. The neurophysiologist José Delgado had carried out similar studies, but in a social setting, published in the 1960s. In his work, Delgado stimulated various brain regions in monkeys as they moved about in their social groups. This was accomplished using transmitted radio signals, so that the animal subject did not have to be restrained and connected to laboratory equipment. He wrote:

> Offensive and defensive responses may be evoked in a single animal, but the most important aspects of aggressive and submissive behavior occur in confrontations among individuals of the same species, which obviously require social situations.
>
> . . . Effects of brain stimulation were more complex and better organized in the free animal than in the animal under restraint. Social situations permitted the study of social activities and also facilitated the expression of evoked behavior and the interpretation of its meaning by observation of the reactions of the group.[8]

In other words, not only did the effects of stimulation depend on the social context—in which, as it happened, the effects were richer and more coherent than in isolation—but Delgado could use the *social responses of the other animals* as indicators of the meaning of the evoked actions of the target subject. This truly social approach, pioneered 3 decades ago, is among the forerunners of the contemporary social view of the brain.

The two paradigms can even alternate in a single experiment, as happens when scientists must step away from the isolated brain paradigm and into the social paradigm in order to interpret the brain activity they are measuring. An example comes from the laboratory of the neurophysiologists Steven Grant and D. Eugene Redmond, who studied the responses of neurons in alert monkeys. The region they studied is called the locus coeruleus, and it is of special interest because it contains neurons that produce catecholamines, adrenalin-like substances known to be important in mood and arousal. They noted that, in general, locus coeruleus neurons fire briskly in response to threatening or unpleasant stimuli, such as toe pinches or threatening gestures. Inconsistent with this general finding, however, was the discovery that locus coeruleus neurons responded to the presentation of a desirable food such as an apple. A previous study had shown that the neurons did not fire when animal subjects received juice by an automated delivery system, which also made it hard to understand why the presentation of apples to the animals caused the neurons to fire.

The researchers explained the paradox by stepping back to analyze the *social* setting of the experiment. They realized that it was the presence of the experimenter with the food that was responsible for the neurons' responses:

> Food presentation by the experimenter could constitute an implied threat of punishment or deprivation, as food consumption by an inferior ranking primate in the presence of a higher ranking one in a macaque social group usually involves a direct or indirect threat of attack as well as the threat that the food may be taken away.[9]

When is the social dimension of brain activity critical, and when can scientists study the brain in social isolation without doing violence to its social nature? Probably, both frameworks should be used side-by-side, and be brought into play to greater or lesser degrees depending on the function being studied. It is unlikely that a simple reflex such as a knee jerk, or an early visual process such as the impact of light on the rods and cones of the retina, requires a social context in order to be understood. At the opposite end, it is almost certainly impossible to understand consciousness or expressive behavior in the absence of a social context. Dreaming, reasoning, and remembering—in other words, many of the most important research topics in cognitive neuroscience—are somewhere in the middle.

Shifts in the way scientists think occur in large part because a new way of thinking is simply more useful than an older way. As we saw, it may be useful for explaining otherwise anomalous research findings, such as cells that fire when faces are seen or when experimenters give apples to monkeys. But a new framework may also allow scientists to integrate their discoveries more successfully with those of researchers in other disciplines. Indeed, researchers in fields such as infant development, primatology, and—of course—sociology have long been occupied with social behavior. These fields had embraced a social as opposed to isolated mind framework for understanding primates, human and nonhuman, long before Kling's lesion studies and Gross's single neuron studies. One of the great benefits of adopting a social framework for studying the primate brain has been the possibility of forming new bridges with other fields. And as neuroscientists continue to move into a social way of thinking, they continue to make contact with a treasure trove of observations and analyses of the mind in social context. In the next section we explore just a sample of the phenomena that are right at the margins of what neuroscientists are currently able to explain—and that we can expect will shortly be within their grasp.

Horizons of the Social Mind

Undoubtedly, one of our most basic social behaviors is our urge for contact. And indeed, anthropological and paleontological evidence indicates that our ancestors evolved in small, cohesive groups.[10] We can thus assume that a host of mechanisms developed to support and maintain a high degree of sociality in our species. Among these would be brain states that cause isolation to be avoided: Indeed, the unpleasant feeling of being an outsider, of "not belonging," can be generated by electrical stimulation of the brain, as we saw in chapter 4. The strongly motivating quality of this social response together with its universality are revealed by the use and effectiveness of ostracism as a punishment in many societies.

There are many cultural mechanisms for stimulating the feeling of belonging through shared physical, affective, and ideational experience. Synchronized group activities such as occur among spectators at large public events, or in certain ensemble performances in which each individual carries out precisely the same routine as the others, are experienced as highly pleasurable by participants. These activities have become ritualized in many cultures as in the various forms of drill-team or synchronized dance. Their purpose may be to generate and express strong feelings of belonging. The human capacity for imitation has parallels in the behavior of both apes and monkeys. It has been suggested that such imitation in nonhuman primates is critical for the transmission of knowledge and skills. Purposeful imitation purely for social pleasure, for the pleasure of being at one with the group, is apparently seen only in human beings. The "contact urge," as the psychologist Géza Révész has theorized, aims at the establishment of a community as an end in itself.[11]

So-called "mob behavior" illustrates how the human need for collective experience may manifest itself in extreme form. In his classic work *The Crowd,* the sociologist Le Bon noted that at a certain phase of organization, the feelings and thoughts of a collectivity turn in an identical direction. This "psychological law of the mental unity of crowds"—as he described it—brings about a lowering of intellectual functions, an intensification of emotional reactions, and on occasion a disregard for personal profit that is reflected in collective acts of heroism and self-sacrifice. Furthermore, crowd psychology creates a readiness to adopt doctrines, explanations, even to endorse shared experiences, which turn out to be illusions on a mass scale. That is, mob conditions appear to facilitate not only a contagion of feelings, but also of ideas and perceptions:

The first perversion of the truth effected by one of the individuals of the gathering is the starting-point of the contagious suggestion. Before St. George appeared on the walls of Jerusalem to all the Crusaders he was certainly perceived in the first instance by one of those present. By dint of suggestion and contagion the miracle signalized by a single person was immediately accepted by all.

Such is always the mechanism of the collective hallucinations so frequent in history—hallucinations which seem to have all the recognized characteristics of authenticity, since they are phenomena observed by thousands of persons.[12]

Mass hysteria is a similar phenomenon. It is characterized by the rapid spread of physical symptoms having no medical basis, a shared—usually irrational—belief regarding their origin and contagious anxiety. For the latter reason, the phenomenon has also been called "hysterical contagion." One such outbreak has been particularly well documented. It began on a day in June in 1962, in a textile mill in a small Southern town. Symptoms of illness were attributed to the bites of an insect believed to have arrived in a cloth shipment from overseas.

The first case was a young woman of 22 who complained of a bite on the Friday before the first big day of the epidemic. Soon afterwards, she fainted. . . . The second case, which occurred on the following Tuesday, was a young woman who worked near the first case. She said she had been bitten the previous week, but she did not report to the doctor until that Tuesday when she complained that she felt "like a balloon ready to burst." On the same day four other women reported to the doctor. The third case passed out soon after having been bitten that afternoon. . . . The fourth case complained not of a bite but of a crawling sensation on her thigh, and she almost passed out. Late that afternoon the fifth and sixth cases occurred when two women became emotionally disturbed and one of them fainted. The next morning the epidemic developed with a rush. Eleven women reported to the medical authorities before noon, and the contagion began to snowball.[13]

Within several days 57 individuals were reported as ill.

The exact precipitating factors of such episodic events as mob behavior and hysterical contagion are difficult to specify in retrospect, and cannot be studied prospectively in a controlled fashion. Several findings that emerged from the study of the textile mill events indicated that there had been a breakdown in organizational structure at the mill when the outbreak began. This suggests contagious behavior may serve to reaffirm the sense of collectivity in groups whose structural cohesion is under strain. In any case, mechanisms for the spread of such behavior must be primitive, for its simpler forms are seen in primates only distantly related to ourselves: Groups of baboons have been observed to pick up rhythmic grunting initiated by one individual; a chorus of such grunting may propagate through the group before eventually dissipating.[14] Human beings do the same thing, but they rationalize it: If I am in a concert hall and hear someone cough, I may suddenly feel as though I too need to cough—and so I do. Perhaps the spread of coughing in a library or silent concert hall derives from an ancient group mechanism for providing affiliative assurance in a group whose members are not otherwise interacting and therefore not assuring each other of their mutual bonds. This seems a better explanation for outbreaks of coughing than the idea that there is just a simultaneous discovery on the part of several people at once of a tickle in their throats—although they may explain it that way to themselves.

For human infants, episodes of shared action in one-on-one encounters serve a very important purpose—they create a conviction on the infant's part that there is a subjective world that it shares with caregivers. How do we know that shared action is important to infants? Researchers have shown that an infant in the 4- to 10-month age range pays special attention when the mother imitates an action it has just performed. Mothers seem to enjoy imitation games too, using them to "teach" shared experience to their babies. The developmental psychologist Ina Uzgiris and her colleagues studied changes in the patterns of mutual imitation between mothers and infants during the first year of life. For younger infants, in the 10-week age group, they found that the mother matched the baby's facial, vocal, or manual actions. As the infants grew older, additional acts such as gaze direction and hand-banging were matched by the mother. For younger infants, it was more often the mother who imitated the baby than the reverse. By the end of the first year, however, both mother and infant matched each other's activity. And by that time, matching activity had become elaborated from simple short episodes to longer, more practiced episodes. Uzgiris speculated that mutual imitation sequences become components of ever-longer scenarios in which mutual understanding comes to be presumed by both partners, because the matched acts have a common meaning. Developmental psychologists Andrew Meltzoff and Alison Gopnik suggested that a primordial sense of kinship, "like me-ness," is the pleasurable result, for both parent and child, of imitation games. All of these observations seem to suggest that the infant's basic faith in a shared world of subjectivity emerges from a matrix of physical interactions.

The intersubjective faith is clearly expressed by around age 1, when infants show by their attempts at communication that they believe

minds can be interfaced with one another through mutually compre-
hensible signals. They first use signals, such as pointing and gaze direction, to establish joint topics of attention with their mother at around 9
months of age. By persisting and repeating their signals when messages
have not been understood, and by timing their gestures to make themselves understood, infants show they believe persons can share understandings. Such a belief in shared understanding is a prerequisite for
creating deliberate exchanges of meaning, such as that which occurs
later in pretend play. Social pretend play involves the active co-construction of a detailed intersubjective world. As a starting framework,
children use their *shared* knowledge of scripts (what happens at din-
nertime; what happens at a birthday party, what happens at the doctor's office) to support extended interactions with peers, with whom
they can then collaboratively construct episodes. All of these findings
outline how infants come to *believe* in a shared world, and how young
children then go on to use shared frameworks for *creating* and *sustaining* social activity.[15]

We can conclude that our species has a predilection for believing in
intersubjectivity—the practices that establish it are carried out by all
normal infants and adults. Does intersubjectivity "really" exist? It
doesn't matter: All that counts is our capacity to believe in it and, with
the collaborative help of those around us, to make it work for us.[16]

We have seen that on some occasions, for reasons we don't fully understand, shared experience takes primitive and even destructive forms
in some human groups, as in mob phenomena and hysterical contagion.
In these cases, the shared experience takes a form that spills over into
the physical domain. Such contagious social phenomena underline the
fragility and contingency of the so-called individual self.[17] They may be
indicators of a primordial condition of pure belonging that, evolutionarily speaking, predated concepts of "self" and "other." Recently, the
neurophysiologist Giacomo Rizzolatti has found neurons in monkeys
that fire both when the monkey carries out certain specific hand motions, and when it views those specific motions being carried out by
someone else. Various neurons of this class, which he terms "mirror
neurons," respond to various motions—but all share the property of
transcending self and other in their representation of action. Based on
preliminary data, it is likely that mirror neurons will also be found for
other gestures, including facial movements. Findings such as these suggest that an archaic kind of sociality, one which does not distinguish self
from other, is woven deeply into the primate brain.[18]

By virtue of having shifted to a social view of the brain, neuroscientists have reached a new threshold. They are beginning to describe

mechanisms that might be responsible for contagious and intersubjective behavior. They are beginning to understand brain specializations for the exquisitely specific social responses that underpin competition, affiliation, play, mating, and parenting. And they are beginning to look into the complexity and importance of communication—not just as the set of statements individuals can make about the world, but as the very framework in which meaning is collaboratively created.

6

Talking Faces

Narratives

Our inborn language capacity is brought to life when we are exposed to the language of our community during infancy and childhood. Before social exposure, language exists only as a kind of abstract potential. This is also true of the concept of person in its social dimension. Our brains have the capacity to generate the concepts of person and social order, but they must take their specific form from exposure to a particular culture. Cultures transmit the content of person and social order in two ways—through *narratives* and *performances*. Let's consider narratives first.

Narratives are inherently public: They are elaborated by individuals in social settings in order to communicate and to be responded to with other narratives.[1] They are about the relations between persons and the social order in the speaker's culture. The function of narrative is to reveal and comment on the language of the social order—that is, on the shoulds, oughts, entitlements, and justifications of everyday life. This definition is consistent with that of the psychologist Jerome Bruner, who maintains, in part, that stories relate to what is morally valued. Bruner also emphasizes that narratives are concerned simultaneously with the subjective world of an individual and with canonical elements of culture—the two dimensions of person first introduced in chapter 1.[2]

The relationship between individual persons and the social order is, therefore, the essence of narrative. Seeing narrative in this way explains why stories about people and their behavior are endlessly fascinating: We, the recipients, are constantly creating and reworking our social worlds, listening to and wielding stories both as inventive forays and as demonstrations. The following fragment of conversation, recorded during a dinner party that included two couples and their children, captures the flavor of everyday narrative.[3]

Beth: What happened?
Ann: Karen has this new house, and it's got all this, like, silvery-gold wallpaper. And Don says—you know, this is the first time we've seen this house, fifty-thousand dollars in Cherry Hill, right?
Beth: Uh-huh?
Ann: Don said, "Did they make you take this wallpaper? Or did you pick it out?" You know, that was like the first bad one.
Don: But I said it so innocuously, you know.
Ann: Yeah, I'm sure they thought it was.

Ann is telling a story to Beth. Explicitly, she is recounting something embarrassing that her husband Don said to Karen. In response to being depicted as the perpetrator of a faux pas, Don offers a mitigation—that his manner, at least, was inoffensive. The story also refers covertly to the tacky décor of the home of a mutual friend, Karen, a décor presumably at odds with the high-status neighborhood of the newly purchased house. In fact, the story is as much about Karen's pretensions to status as it is about Don's faux pas. Ann's poke at these pretensions is carried out with social skill, which is to say, her deprecation of Karen is expressed indirectly.

A great deal of shared understanding must exist in order for such an exchange to take place and make sense to the participants. Presumably, all the adults in this conversation "got" what Ann was saying about Karen's house. They understood that Karen's claim to social status—which Ann was challenging by her description of the wallpaper—was as much the topic of the story as Don's gaffe. Such claims to status and their contestation may form a universal topical category in everyday narrative. Unlike such universal aspects of social order, however, other social categories belong only to a particular culture. An example is what it means to be a "wife," which is in some ways the same and in some ways different from culture to culture and from epoch to epoch. Others are more local still: the necessary acts and attitudes of a "hostess" depend on whether a child's birthday party or a wedding reception is the context. Although some social categories become objects of struggle between political factions within a single society (a contemporary example is the status of domestic animals as objects of moral concern), most categories are part of our mental landscape. We take them as simple facts and are thereby enabled to carry out interactions with others with relative ease. And this is precisely what acculturation accomplishes: through narratives and performances (we take up the latter in the next section), it turns arbitrary social categories into a felt reality for participants.

Why are narratives so influential? Belonging is a primary human motivation: In order to belong, individuals adopt and use the narratives that surround them. Thus, the group's narratives organize the thought of its members, specifying the categories of their perceptions, especially perceptions regarding persons. The domain of social meanings conveyed by acts and stories is like a language in that it is a network of interdependent meanings taken up by children from those around them. In this way, children become members of a social order.

Following Richard Dawkins, Daniel Dennett calls the smallest units of such stories "memes." Memes, according to Dennett, are cultural ideas (such as Impressionism, chess, vendetta, wearing clothes) that flow from brain to brain, where they behave like parasites, replicating and spreading to new host brains competitively. We can expand this idea to note that, not only small units, but whole networks of meaning used by the group (and each of the elements in the preceding list exists in a web of related concepts) are taken up by individuals. Although this spread takes place so quickly and effectively that it indeed invites comparison to an invasion, let's see if we can describe it in more mundane, empirical terms. It arises through the simple act of imitation, the most basic kind of social participation.

The developmental psychologist John Dore describes the earliest stages of acquisition of complex social narratives by a 2-year-old child, seeing them as "reenvoicements" of her parents' talk. His research illustrates how discourse genres are first co-constructed with more fully socialized agents of language—namely, parents. Dore concludes that it is not only the child's social talk, but her very thinking that reflects the voices of others. Acquiring social forms seems to be a special talent of the human species, for adults and children alike.[4] There is an exception though: Autistic people do not produce narratives. This makes sense in light of the idea that autistic individuals do not achieve the concept of person—for that is what narratives are all about.[5]

Usually, however, cultural learning determines how we construct the personhood of our fellow beings. We can use Robinson Crusoe's fictional experience at the moment of sighting the footprint in the sand as an example. Consider the physical feature that Crusoe saw, the footprint. Endowed by Defoe with a normal brain that automatically generated the concept of person from lower level physical features, Crusoe did not pause to consider what the footprint betokened. Inferring the recent presence of a foot, he could only feel the presence of a being with a mental life. But what kind of being? A product of his culture, Crusoe first decided it must be the devil, and held a rather lengthy debate with himself for and against this idea, before discarding it as inconsistent with "all the notions we usually entertain of the subtility of the devil" (p.205).

By providing categories and concepts, the narratives of eighteenth century Europe had organized this fictional character's experience, causing the otherwise ambiguous footprint to be experienced as a manifestation of the devil (a person with a definite place in the moral social order). We will consider the workings of the acculturation process in detail in chapter 7. As we will see, it is through acculturation that events in the world come to be understood in a particular way and their meanings become "obvious." We must suppose that the human drive to participate in collective life through contagion, imitation, and identification causes us to adopt the speeches and practices typical of our society. Belief follows from participation: Thus, the narratives and meanings we use in order to belong are also our own.

Before leaving narrative, we will note one more of its characteristics. The relationships between persons and the social order are expressed in the language of reasons rather than in the language of causes. What is the distinction between reasons and causes? Causes belong to the world of natural science. Scientific accounts state, for example, that "ice floats *because* it is less dense than liquid water." Narratives, on the other hand, invoke reasons. For example, "As a baby, Frederick was accidentally apprenticed to pirates. When he grew up they would not release him *because* he was indentured until age 21, but was born on the last day of February in a leap year." The relationship between reasons and causes is of interest to philosophers: As Frederick's remaining physically on board the pirate ship shows, human *reasons* seem to produce physical effects— just like causes.[6] But reasons belong to the language of the social order, whereas causes belong to the language of natural science.

Performances

Narratives are informative; conversations are performative. Although narratives—using the vocabulary of reasons and "shoulds"—educate us about what it means to be a particular kind of person in our culture, conversations are where personhood is exercised in the here and now. In conversation, persons mark their momentary status in the social order by deploying signs. By their speech or nonverbally, they may enact deference or authority, femaleness or maleness, unconventionality or ordinariness.[7] The stream of signs in here-and-now, face-to-face interactions is rapid and complex. Roles such as speaker and listener are or-chestrated by participants through collective structuring of these streams. In a sense, conversations need not be verbal at all, but may consist of *any* array of publicly intelligible signs. The social psycholo-gist Rom Harré has considered performative conversations to have a more extended form: They can be "any flow of interactions brought about through the use of a public semiotic system, such as that in-volved in the meaningful flying of flags, the wearing of uniforms, ball-room dancing."[8] The following passage from a novel is telling:

> When she had resolved to go down, she prepared herself by some little acts which might seem mere folly to a hard onlooker; they were her way of expressing to all spectators visible or invisible that she had begun a new life in which she embraced humiliation. She took off all her ornaments and put on a plain black gown, and instead of wearing her much-adorned cap and large bows of hair, she brushed her hair down and put on a plain bonnet-cap, which made her look suddenly like an early Methodist. . . .
> He burst out crying and they cried together, she sitting at his side. They could not yet speak to each other of the shame which she was bearing with him, or of the acts which had brought it down on them. His confession was silent, and her promise of faithfulness was silent.[9]

This excerpt from the novel *Middlemarch* shows that performative communications need not be linguistic at all. It depicts the actions of a Mrs. Bulstrode, who has just learned that her husband, previously an individual of high social standing, has become disgraced. The gossip-ing goodwives of Middlemarch had speculated among themselves, in preceding pages, as to what Mrs. Bulstrode's course of action would be when she found out what had happened: Most were of the opinion that she would be within her rights to leave her husband. By her dress and actions, however, Mrs. Bulstrode signals both her adoption of her husband's fallen status, and her commitment to a particular construc-tion of the role of wife. The two main themes of the novel, social hier-archy and marriage, are brought to a remarkable intersection at this point, one made especially dramatic by the absence of spoken words. Like all great narratives, the tale as a whole is compelling precisely be-cause it is about *the relationship between individual persons and the so-cial order*. We see in this excerpt how Mrs. Bulstrode "performed" a wifely role, which at the same time was an individual act of choosing.

Faces in Action

Although social performances may consist entirely of nonverbal signs, as in the literary example above, they usually take the form of integrated packets of speech, facial gestures, and vocal intonation—in other words, everyday "talk." The neurolinguists Richard Patry and Jean-Luc Nespoulous observed:

> All the steps involved in conversation require close attention of each participant to the other(s) in order to give and receive information; moreover, this information is not always expressed through verbal channels alone, but also by mimicry, gestures, eye movements, or posture, for example. Thus, conversation is certainly the linguistic context in which the relation between signs and users finds it fullest extension.[10]

The face-to-face encounter, in other words, is richly performative. Prior to the invention of insignias and ceremonies, in our evolution, prolonged face-to-face encounters must have been the first field in which humans displayed and exchanged signals, the ground on which they tested, cajoled, and appeased one another while other members of the group looked on. Conversation begins with faces.

Facial expressions are imperative signals for all primates. The neural equipment that generates and perceives these expressions is far older than the human species. But the human brain has brought facial displays under a high degree of control to produce subtly modulated streams of signals. These signals, accompanied by words, are publicly exchanged in the breathtakingly rapid pas de deux of conversation. Although in this chapter we will concentrate primarily on the role of the face in conversation, other bodily gestures, voice intonation, and non-word sounds are also important ingredients.[11] A complete account of conversation would include a description of how the brain orchestrates all these features of "talk." Here, though, we look in detail at how faces evolved to become the vehicles of conversation.

Conversation is easy for us to "do," so at first it might seem that it would also be easy to understand. But when we look at it from the outside, simple conversation becomes a feat that calls for quite a bit of explaining. Let's put ourselves in a naive position, approaching conversation as novices rather than as the experts we are.

Oddly enough, conversation may have evolved from primate social grooming, the activity of brushing and picking through the fur of other animals in one's group. Grooming is widespread in primate species and much time is devoted to it. The likelihood of its being engaged in by any pair or group of individuals is dependent on factors such as the social rank and relationship of the participants, as well as social contexts such as previous aggression or the possibility of mating. As in human conversation, partners may alternate roles of giver and receiver. Although grooming confers some survival value because parasites are being removed, and conversation may confer some survival value by the transmission of information, they are time-consuming far beyond the survival value they may confer. The primary purpose of both grooming and conversation is to maintain and update social bonds. All these similarities suggest conversation is evolutionarily related to the mutual grooming engaged in by apes and monkeys.[12]

Conversation appears to be enjoyed universally in human groups. It is a highly structured, cooperative enterprise that requires the active participation of listeners as well as speakers. In English-speaking communities, where conversation has been most extensively studied, it is characterized by specific procedures for turn-taking, lack of prespecification of content, indeterminateness of the number of turns per participant, and conventions for opening and closing.[13] Other speech events, such as debates, lectures, and panel discussions, are not considered conversations because they possess different properties. Speech events having the properties of conversation are recognized as the social object "conversation" by members. That this recognition is *given* becomes apparent in situations in which interlocutors supply a context that accounts for and excuses deviations from convention—for example, when we converse with a very young child or a disorganized schizophrenic. In such cases, the conventional rule-using participant in effect provides a dispensation to the other participant, such that the event may still be held to be a "conversation." Under normal circumstances, though, a conversation's form is created by coordinated activity on the part of all parties, activity that is highly constrained by complex—if tacit—rules.

Much of what is communicated therefore, both verbally and nonverbally, is information regarding the structure of the conversation itself. Speakers and listeners alike continually emit signals of the states of their participation as role players. They behave at all times as though they are accountable to others present for contributing to the moment-to-moment weaving of the interactive fabric. This behavior is the focus of a branch of sociology called "conversation analysis." The techniques of conversation analysis were applied by Charles Goodwin to the short dinner table "story" that was introduced above as an example of everyday narrative. Let's return to it. The participants in this conversation were two couples seated with their children at a dinner that was being videotaped. One couple, Ann and Don, are guests; John and Beth are hosts. Ann is recounting that she and Don had a difficult weekend. She relates to Beth what Don said about the wallpaper in Karen's new house.

Figure 6.1 presents one of Goodwin's simplified transcripts of the wallpaper story. In addition to documenting the words, it encodes

```
 4   Beth:   What h ⌐appened.
 5   Ann:         ⌊Karen has this new hou: se. en it's got
 6           all this like- (0.2) ssilvery : : g-go:ld
 7           wwa:llpaper, •hh (h)en D(h) o (h)n sa(h)ys,
 8           y'know this's th'firs'time we've seen this
 9           house.=Fifty five thousn dollars in Cherry
10           Hill.=Right?
11                   (0.4)
12   Beth:   Uh hu: h?
13   Ann:    Do(h)n said.  (0.3) dih-did they ma: ke you take
14           this ⌐wa(h)llpa(h)p(h)er? er(h)di ⌐dju  pi (h) ck⌐
15   Beth:        ⌊hh!                         ⌊Ahh huh huh⌊
16   Ann:    =⌐⌐i(h)t  ou(h)t.
17   Beth:    ⌊⌊huh huh huh  ⌐huh
18   Don:                    ⌊ Uhh hih huh huh ⌐h
19   Ann:                                     ⌊ UHWOOghghHHH!=
20   Ann:    =Y'kno(h)w that wz ⌐like the firs' bad one.
21   Beth:                      ⌊ Uh :oh wo: :w hh
22                   (0.2)
23   Don:    But I said it so innocuously y'know.
24   Ann:    Yeh I'm sure they thought it wz- hnh hnh!
```

Figure 6.1　Transcript fragment. *From Structures of Social Action: Studies in Conversation Analysis*, pp. 225–226 by C. Goodwin, 1984, Cambridge, UK: Cambridge University Press. Copyright © Maison de Sciences de l'Hommes and Cambridge University Press. Reprinted with the permission of Cambridge University Press.

various nonlinguistic sounds, pause durations, and the degree to which turns overlap. Although speakers and listeners register and respond to such features in their interactions—as an analysis of conversational episodes demonstrates—these cues are exceedingly difficult to notice consciously. To accurately record sounds, pauses, and turn overlaps in natural conversation requires extensive experience and the patience to listen over and over again to taped segments as short as 1 second in duration. To record shifts in gaze, head nods, and facial expressions requires an equally painstaking dissection of the videotaped record. But once the data is carefully sifted in this way, it reveals something counterintuitive: although everyday talk may feel effortless, participants actually are responding and adjusting to one another continuously, with lightning speed, and on several channels at the same time. As we peer through the lens of Goodwin's analysis, we will begin to discover just how densely interactive the brief wallpaper conversation was.

Among the nonverbal signals Goodwin transcribed were "laugh tokens," for which he used the symbol (h). Laugh tokens are small, voiced exhalations during speech by means of which the speaker comments, paralinguistically, that *this* is the funny part, and by which he or she implicitly invites listeners to laugh. As Goodwin puts it, by producing such sounds the speaker is making relevant particular types of subsequent action by recipients of the story as it unfolds. These sounds also give information about the structure of what is being said. By the distribution of laugh tokens during her speech, Ann demarcates segments of her talk, which include a background, a climax, and a section of background information embedded disjunctively within the climax ("this is the first time . . . fifty-thousand dollars in Cherry Hill").

It is risky business for a speaker to take her listeners on a detour during the climax of a story. Because Ann's placing of the parenthetic "Cherry Hill" information within the climax of the story posed a problem for the listeners in their roles as interactants, their responses to this disjunctive element in the story were carefully analyzed. For example, Beth was the addressed recipient. The videotape record showed that Beth changed her orientation to Ann as the climax of the story began ("and Don says—"), leaning toward her and thereby signaling she was treating this section of the story differently from the background that had just preceded it. At that point, however, Ann began her parenthesis. Marking her awareness that this was not after all the climax, Beth withdrew her gaze from Ann as Ann reached the word "thousand." Ann therefore appended an explicit request for a display of coparticipation, the question, "Right?" Beth did not produce a response for four-tenths of a second—a significant duration in the swift time scales of human conversation—but then indicated her participation by saying, "Uh-huh?" Having received this response, Ann returned immediately to the climax segment of the story.

Don, the principal character of the story, was seated next to Ann during the telling. Don behaved as though his task was to arrange his behavior at the climax of the story so that he would be available for the story-relevant scrutiny it would receive from the others present. During the parts of the story that were leading up to his reported speech, he directed his face toward the listeners, but kept his eyes downcast and covered his mouth with his hand. Goodwin noted:

> This position, somewhat like that of an actor who has moved to the wings but is not yet on stage, appears transitional. It places the party who adopts it in a position that is relevant to upcoming events in the sequence of talk (i.e., his face is available for story-relevant scrutiny by the others present) but the party adopting this position is not yet displaying full engagement with his coparticipants.[14]

This interpretation of Don's posture is borne out by the fact that, when Ann entered the parenthesis, he moved his head to the side, shifting his gaze to a ladle of soup. There he kept his gaze until the parenthesis ended. At "Don said" he returned his face to the focus of the conversation and placed his hand at his mouth in the same position as before the start of the parenthesis. As the story approached the climax phrase "pick it out," he was producing an escalating smile, culminating in a sharp head movement that coincided with Ann's rush of laugh tokens. At the punchline, everyone at the table who was looking at someone, was looking at Don, whose behavior, especially his face, was now "arranged" for just this public observation.

John, the nonaddressed recipient of the story, had the task (so to speak) of being appreciative when the punchline arrived. Throughout the story he was apparently attending to the process of serving himself soup; however, analysis of the videotape revealed that even his ladling movements were structured around the storyteller's activities. When Ann signaled, by her laugh tokens, that the climax of the story was approaching, John stopped ladling, and held the ladle still in midair. When it became apparent that a parenthesis was underway, he resumed ladling. When the punchline actually came, he had a full ladle, but dropped it back into the bowl again, and looked at Don. John, by his activities with the ladle, marked parts of Ann's story as background, where other activities such as eating can legitimately be done, and climax, where they cannot.

This is an ordinary, everyday bit of conversation. Until one looks closely, it is not obvious how much careful, collaborative work goes into sustaining conversation as a structured activity. Although we think of conversation as having to do with words, much of what is achieved in conversation has little to do with linguistic content. It consists mostly of nonlinguistic role-playing and signals to others regarding what their expected role behavior is to be. Although we ordinarily regard words and sentences as memorable, rather than patterns of gazes and smiles, words and sentences are but one layer of an integrated, multilayer message.[15] The words, on the one hand, and the nonverbal activity, on the other, form a whole—like the lyrics and melody of a well-written song. Facial gestures, for example, are used extensively to coordinate conversation. Let's turn to them now.

The neuropsychologist William Rinn wrote:

> Although most observers would agree that facial behavior plays an important role in communication, few appreciate the immense complexity and richness of the messages conveyed . . . the first thing one is struck with is the surprising frequency of facial gestures. For many subjects, the face and head are almost constantly generating expressions and gestures.[16]

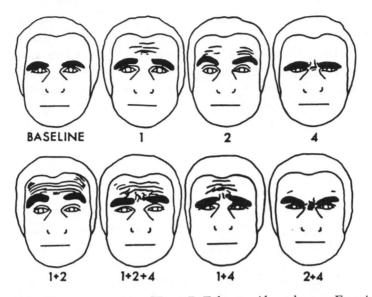

BASELINE   1   2   4

1+2   1+2+4   1+4   2+4

Figure 6.2   Brow movements. [From P. Eckman. About brows: Emotional and conversational signals. In J. Aschoof, M. von Cranach, K. Foppa, W. Lepenies, and D. Ploog (eds.) *Human Ethology: Claims and Limits of a New Discipline* (p. 174) 1979, Cambridge, UK: Cambridge University Press. Copyright © 1979 by Cambridge University Press. Reprinted with permission of Cambridge University Press.]

Yet, despite this promising abundance of expressiveness in conversation, the psychologist Paul Ekman notes, "Compared to the emotional expressions, relatively little is known about conversational signals. We do not know of any quantitative studies of these actions."[17]

Perhaps facial gestures in conversation have not been the subject of much empirical study because their fleetingness makes them technically difficult to detect, and their abundance is time-consuming to describe. Nevertheless, Ekman made some qualitative observations regarding the role of eyebrow motions in conversations. He first categorized brow movements into seven different displays, each formed by the action of different muscles or combinations of muscles (see Figure 6.2). In conversation, as opposed to emotional expression, Ekman found that two brow configurations, a combination of actions 1 and 2, and action 4, occurred frequently. He speculated that these are used in conversation both because they are easiest to perform, and because they are easiest to detect, being at the extremes of movement (from raised high to lowered and drawn together).

He then listed the functions that brow movements served in conversation. For speakers, brow movements can add emphasis to speech, coinciding with primary voice stress or other voiced forms of emphasis; they can be used to add meaning at the end of a clause, both marking the clause and conveying an attitude such as exclamation, doubt, or difficulty about the content of the clause; they can be used to indicate a question; and they can be used to "hold the floor" while the speaker searches for a word. Listeners use brow motions to signal either agreement, disbelief, or incredulity. Finally, brow motions can be used as signals in the absence of speech, as in the "flash" (raised brows) that can indicate greeting, the combination of raised brows and dropped jaw that signals mock astonishment, and so forth.[18]

The psychologist Nicole Chovil carried out a careful quantitative study of how facial displays work in conjunction with verbal content.[19] In her study, pairs of undergraduate volunteer subjects who did not know each other previously were introduced to one another and given several topics for discussion. They could talk about planning a nutritional meal using foods they disliked; they could retell a conversation that involved a minor conflict between themselves and another person; and they could tell about a close-call or "near miss" situation that they had experienced or heard about. They conversed spontaneously in pairs for 5 minutes on each topic while being videotaped.

Chovil defined facial displays as "movement or change in one or more areas of the face (i.e., brows, eyes, nose, mouth)" (p. 56). For practical reasons, she excluded smiles because they occurred so frequently, sometimes throughout whole conversations. The facial displays she studied consisted of "one or more actions such as eyebrow raising or lowering, eyes widening or squinting, nose wrinkling, upper lip raises, mouth corners pulled back or down, etc." (pp. 56–57). For every facial display in the recorded conversations, a description of the facial action and the verbal context in which it occurred was noted. She noted who made the display (speaker or listener); what kind of information was conveyed (syntactic, semantic, or nonlinguistic); and whether the information in the display was independent of or redundant with the verbal content.

Chovil found that the largest number of facial movements were used by speakers to mark structural aspects of an utterance, rather than meaning. Twenty-seven percent of the facial displays were syntactic. They marked stress on particular words or clauses, were connected with syntactic aspects of utterances, or were connected with organizational structure, such as topics. Examples of these included movements of the eyebrows for emphasis, to indicate questions, and to "underline" phrases.

The next most common use of facial gesture by speakers was as an illustrator. The information conveyed by a facial illustrator is at least partly redundant with the information being given by the verbal content. Portrayal is one type of illustration. Eyebrow raising might be used to indicate that a portrayal was taking place, as in the following example in which the content of a past conversation was marked for the listener (brackets correspond to duration of raised eyebrows): "and I said [Is there any need to talk to me like that?]" (p. 77).

Finally, speakers used facial movements to make communications that commented on their own verbal utterance, adding information not present in the utterance. Examples are facial movements showing the speaker's stance with respect to his own verbalization (e.g., showing disgust) or indications of sarcasm or of a joke.

Listeners in this study also used facial displays actively. The most frequent use of facial gestures by listeners was to communicate to the speaker that the listener was attending to what was being said. Chovil's analysis revealed that these typically consisted of eyebrow raises, mouth corners turned down, eyes closed, or lips pressed. Her results show how extensively facial signaling is called on to structure everyday conversation.

With the shift to a social perspective on the brain, scientists have begun to focus on the evolutionary origins of paralinguistic gestures, those gestures that add information to the overall message using nonverbal channels. Expressive faces pose a problem, however. Classically, psychologists have contrasted "emotional" expression—with its connotations of irrationality and involuntariness—with linguistic expression, which is associated with rationality and voluntary control. As we've seen, facial gestures that accompany conversation seem to be related to emotional expressiveness, for they use the same medium—the face; but they also seem to be related to language, for they add information about syntactic structure and about the speech they accompany. Do they belong to expression—in the sense that we connect expressions with feelings—or to language? Let's look at the evidence.

Brains and Face-to-Face Communication

We saw in chapter 4 that primates shifted in the course of evolution from a reliance on olfaction (the sense of smell) to a reliance on visual signaling. In the process, the muscles of their faces were rearranged to produce a rich variety of movements that could be visually communicated: the expressions. On the perceptual side, brain structures that had previously served olfaction were adapted to read visual signals instead.

To trace the evolution of the expressive face, it is useful to compare different primates with one another. Within the primate order, there are several major subdivisions. The prosimians—including the lemurs, tarsiers, and galagos—make up one major subdivision; the other is the anthropoid division, containing New World and Old World monkeys, apes, and humans. The prosimians are considered to be more ancestral (more primitive) than the anthropoid primates. Some of the prosimians, like the insectivores from which they evolved, rely on olfaction; some rely on vision. Monkeys, apes, and humans, in contrast, are fully reliant on vision as a sensory modality.

Whereas primitive primates possess nonmobile upper lips bound to the underlying bone of the upper jaw (similar to those of dogs, for example), an adaptation apparently occurred in other primates, giving rise to the nonattached upper lip. Mobile upper lips are a feature shared by humans, tarsiers, monkeys, and apes. John Allman and Eve-Lynn McGuinness noted that primates with mobile upper lips (called the "haplorhine" primates) tend to live in more complex social groups than do those with nonmobile lips, and to rely in general on vision, rather than on olfaction, for social communication. A reliance on vision and a freeing of facial musculature for use in facial expression seem to have gone hand in hand. The researchers put it this way, "As complex systems of social organization evolved in haplorhine primates, social communication was increasingly mediated by the visual channel at the expense of the olfactory channel."[20] For visual communication, the face is the transmitter.

What makes the face move? A number of facial muscles around the mouth and eyes are innervated by what is known as the facial nerve, or seventh cranial nerve. (The brain's cranial nerves originate in a region of the brain just above the spinal cord called the brainstem.) The function of this nerve, Rinn noted, "is not to perform operations on the environment, but to arrange the facial features in meaningful configurations."[21] The other cranial nerves control many involuntary, stereotyped actions, such as those involved in breathing, coughing, and vomiting. Neural activity originating in an area of the brain known as the basal ganglia can in turn cause the facial nerve to move the face's muscles. Because the face is used expressively in both humans and monkeys, it is probable that this arrangement was in place by the time the common ancestor of humans and nonhuman primates appeared.

Charles Darwin and the researchers who followed him have been more interested in the so-called involuntary facial expressions because they have been thought to be more expressive than voluntary expressions. According to Darwin:

> When movements, associated through habit with certain states of the mind, are partially repressed by the will, the strictly involuntary muscles, as well as those which are least under the separate control of the will, are liable still to act; and their action is often highly expressive. Conversely, when the will is temporarily or permanently weakened, the voluntary muscles fail before the involuntary.[22]

It would be tempting to say that evolutionarily older expressive patterns are produced involuntarily, whereas their socially harnessed, conversational versions are produced voluntarily. Then we could assign involuntary expressions to more ancient brain systems, and look for the mechanisms of voluntary expression in more recently evolved brain structures. But does this dichotomy hold up?

At first it would seem so. Michael Gazzaniga and Charlotte Smylie studied individuals who had undergone commissurotomies—"split brain" patients. Patients who have had this surgery are unable to transfer information between the two hemispheres of the brain. In such individuals, the distinct abilities of the right and left hemispheres can be studied, free from influence by the other side. On a screen in front of the patients, the researchers presented pictures of facial expressions to be imitated, in such a way that they could be seen by only one eye at a time, thus "addressing" the command to only one hemisphere. They videotaped the patients' faces both during this task, and during spontaneous conversation with an experimenter. Because the pathways from the brain motor neurons to the various muscles of the face are known, and because they could analyze the movements of the patients' faces in detail, the researchers were able to infer which hemisphere was active in causing facial movements. Gazzaniga and Smylie found that the patients could not use their right hemispheres to produce facial expressions on command, but that they did use the right equally with the left in producing the facial expressions that occur in conversation.[23] This important observation argues that different mechanisms are responsible for the facial expressions occurring in natural face-to-face encounters than for the kind of facial expressions we make on purpose. Similarly, some patients with neurologic injuries may be unable to smile when asked to by their doctors, but may smile spontaneously at a joke someone has told them, again demonstrating that expressions constructed purposely and expressions produced in response to natural social cues seem to be separately controlled. Because of the contrast with expressions made "to order," expressions in natural face-to-face encounters have been called involuntary—a designation that unfortunately connotes a kind of formless eruption of pure expressiveness. Certainly there are genuine distinctions to be made between purposely constructed expressions and naturally occurring ones: Purposely constructed smiles in social situations differ from their spontaneous counterparts in being more asymmetric. (Strikingly, however, observers usually do not discern the difference between felt and false smiles without special training.[24] If there is an evolutionary advantage to being able to make a facial expression on purpose, it would depend on the expression's being perceived as bona fide. Apparently, false smiles are so perceived.) Nevertheless, even the expressions we normally associate with pure, involuntary emotion are not as simple or involuntary as people often assume. For example, the psychologist Robert Provine conducted a study of laughter by observing small groups of students socializing spontaneously on a college campus. He found that laughter occurred at the end of complete phrases or questions *over 99% of the time.*[25] In only 8 of 1,200 laugh episodes did the speaker interrupt a phrase with laughter, and in *none* of the 1200 episodes was a phrase interrupted with laughter by a listener. It would not make sense to interpret laughter under these conditions as being an involuntary expression of joy, unless one argues that joy is occasioned by the end of a clause. Instead, laughter in everyday conversation apparently serves as a controllable signal both of speaker–listener relations and turn boundaries.

Likewise, naturally occurring human facial expressions defy the simple voluntary versus involuntary distinction. The sequences of facial expressions that unfold during social interactions are both highly constrained by the interactional context—as Chovil and Ekman showed—and produced automatically without conscious planning. They are neither willed performances nor socially unconscious discharges of raw feeling. In fact, the characteristics of facial expressions in normal interactions should make us question the usefulness of the voluntary/involuntary categorization of expression. Instead, to understand brain mechanisms of face-to-face interaction, we should focus on the fact that humans have retained an ancient ability to generate facial expressions, and added to it a capacity for exquisite control. In this way, expressive movements such as those of the eyebrows and corners of the mouth can double as paralinguistic signals that are emitted in rapid and subtle combinations. This trick, adding layers of control onto preexisting capacities, is common in evolution.

How are expressive movements of the face able to be so finely, yet so automatically, controlled? To answer this question, we turn to the part of the brain that is active during fine movements of the muscles, the motor cortex. Figure 6.3 shows what is called "the motor strip homunculus"—*homunculus*, from Latin, for "little man." A cross section

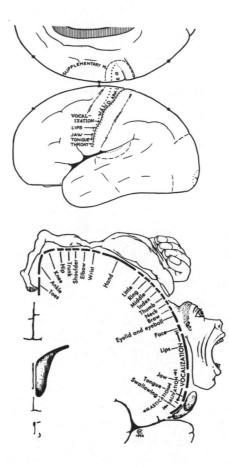

Figure 6.3. (Top) Side view of human brain (front of brain points left). The cell bodies of neurons whose activity causes movement of parts of the body, are organized in a maplike fashion in the cortex of the lateral side (outside) of the brain, a map that extends over the top and into the medial side (inside) of the hemisphere. "Throat," "tongue," "jaw," and so on designate the sites in which neurons causing movements in those parts are found. (From Penfield, W., Roberts, L., Speech and Brain Mechanisms. Copyright © renewed 1959 by Princeton University Press. Reproduced by permission of Princeton University Press.), p. 200.

(Below) A crossection of one hemisphere, taken at the level of the motor strip shown above. Here, instead of the words "throat," "tongue," and "jaw," pictures of the various body parts are shown, their size proportional to the amount of neural tissue that is dedicated to their movements. Both hemispheres have the same motor organization. (Reproduced with the permission of Simon & Schuster, Inc. from *The Cerebral Cortex of Man* by Wilder Penfield and Theodore Rasmussen. Copyright © 1950 by Macmillan Publishing Company; copyright © 1978 by Theodore Rasmussen.), p. 57.

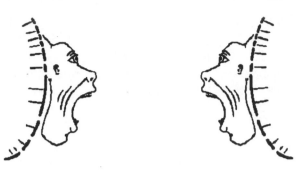

Figure 6.4. The face regions of the motor strip homunculi shown in Figure 6.3, fancifully depicted as if "talking" to one another. (Adapted with the permission of Simon & Schuster, Inc. from *The Cerebral Cortex of Man* by Wilder Penfield and Theodore Rasmussen. Copyright © 1950 by Macmillan Publishing Company; copyright © 1978 by Theodore Rasmussen.)

of the frontal lobe of one side of the brain, at the level of the primary motor cortex, contains an organized map of the body parts that its neurons control (a cross section on the other side contains a map of the same appearance). A representation of the body parts controlled by these neurons, drawn in proportion to the amount of cortex dedicated to each part, gives rise to this odd, but orderly depiction of the body. The feet, legs, and trunk are controlled by cortical tissue at the top of the brain, dipping into the space where the two hemispheres join. The representations of the hand, the face, and the tongue are disproportionately large, in comparison to the legs and trunk. This reflects the degree of fine motor control used to manage the hands and face, and especially the mouth, in humans.

We know that the cortex has great flexibility: Learning complex routines is impossible without motor cortex. Perhaps so much human cortex is devoted to representing face movement because we have to *learn*, through social practice, how people in our native culture deploy expressions. This skill is not optional. It is essential for us to wield facial expressions in accordance with learned rules because our ability to participate in the exchange of signs that makes us members of our social group depends on it. Every human being must learn not one but two systems of facial movement. The first is paralinguistic display, the deployment of facial movements in accordance with cultural rules, which adds information to the verbal message. The second is the use of mouth muscles to articulate speech. One might fancifully say that the homunculus, little though he may be, is a *big* talker (see Figure 6.4), judging by how much motor cortex is dedicated to his mouth! He is indeed *Homo loquens*.[26]

There is another brain region that is critical for normal conversation. The prefrontal cortex has increased markedly in size during primate evolution. The dorsolateral prefrontal regions of the primate frontal lobes are believed to play an important role in working memory, planning, and interference control, key elements of the temporal organization of behavior. It has been shown that there are neurons that respond selectively to the sight of faces in the dorsolateral and prearcuate prefrontal cortices of monkeys. Quite possibly, these frontal lobe structures play a role in high-level aspects of temporally organized social behavior. Indeed, it is difficult to imagine how an everyday face-to-face conversation could be carried out without each participant's having many possible responses in readiness, and continuously updating plans for appropriate responses in light of the unfolding sequence of social signals directed at him or her. Furthermore, participants must be able to emit their own gestures and utterances rapidly and in correct order, even at the same time as they are updating their plans in light of social feedback.

In support of a role for the frontal lobes in organizing conversation, researchers have found that people who suffer lesions of the right frontal cortex do not have problems with language per se but do have problems using it appropriately in social settings. The neurologists Michael Alexander, D. Frank Benson, and Donald Stuss noticed that such patients can't use or understand analogies or irony and that their speech is often tangential or rambling. They don't draw the normal inferences from others' statements—and their own discourse is correspondingly literal and blunt. They also are inattentive to social context and fail to appreciate the impact of their utterances on others.[27] What these patients demonstrate is that socially appropriate conversation, an activity that demands deft analysis of context from moment to moment, is critically dependent on the frontal lobes. Apparently, the prolonged face-to-face encounters typical of our species place considerable demands on working memory—a type of memory for which prefrontal cortex is critical. It is tempting to speculate, therefore, that face-to-face interactions have been a driving force in the evolutionary expansion of our frontal lobes.

To summarize, we have seen that "talk" bears the hallmarks of its descent from facial signaling, and its precursor olfactory signaling. Darwin wrote truly when he said, "The movements of expression give vividness and energy to our spoken words."[28] Expressive displays are attention-getters because our brains are wired to respond to them. But, like tigers in a circus act, they can be made to perform in a constrained and orchestrated fashion. This is the trick our brains have perfected:

The face is the center ring—all eyes are on it. And when we see facial displays, we register them in evolutionarily old brain networks that include structures such as the amygdala. As we learned in chapter 4, these networks are set to trigger behavioral dispositions appropriate to the social situations in which primates have commonly found themselves throughout their history. Building on this basic equipment, with our modern capacity to create culture we generate new situations, new contexts, and new responses through our talk. The humble one-act show for which the face was the primordial center ring has spread out to fill the universe.

Our description of the social brain is now complete. We have taken a close look at face-to-face interaction—the humble loom that ceaselessly weaves the fabric of culture. We now venture out into the remarkable worlds we create.

7

Worlds We Create

The Social Self

We saw in the first four chapters that our brains attribute a locus of subjectivity to faces and bodies, endowing them with mental life, a key dimension of the concept of person. In the last chapter we saw how the relationship between persons and the social order is continuously invented and reworked in narratives and how our brains have evolved to carry out the sophisticated face-to-face performance known as "talk." Thus, we are adapted not only to form the concept of person, but also as receptacles both for communal stories and for performances of what it means to be a person—what a person in one's culture or one's family should do, think, and say. Moreover, we are highly flexible in this regard, even eager to redefine ourselves and each other through our interactions.

The brain's social functions are relatively new to neuroscience. In contrast, the idea that people make social realities through their interactions has long been articulated by philosophers and workers in the social sciences. Some of these thinkers have even proposed that the concept of self is a purely social creation. Does our experience of having a subjective locus of experience—a self—come from our own individual brains? Or does it arise from our participation in a socially constructed universe in which the inhabitants believe in "selves"?

In our survey of the answers that social psychologists have given to these questions, we begin with George Herbert Mead, whose theories, known as "symbolic interactionism," were developed in the early decades of this century.[1] Mead pioneered a thoroughly social theory of the human mind. Meanings, he said, arise in social interaction. He believed that signals directed at others, such as words and gestures, derive their meanings from the utterer's awareness of the reactions the word calls forth inside himself. This awareness betokens the fact that the word is not merely a tool for directing the actions of others, but is instead something with a public meaning, a reaction called forth in all who hear it.

The idea is not easy to understand and can perhaps be made clearer by using one of Mead's own examples. "Property" is shorthand for an organized set of attitudes common to all members of a community. The set includes an attitude of controlling one's own property and of respecting the property of others. What makes society possible is the fact that when a person says, "This is my property," the statement evokes the proper set of responses in all other members of the community. Mead contrasts this social understanding of "property" with the attitude a dog may have for a bone:

> A dog will fight any other dog trying to take the bone. The dog is not taking the attitude of the other dog. A man who says "This is my property" is taking an attitude of the other person. The man is appealing to his rights because he is able to take the attitude which everybody else in the group has with reference to property, thus arousing in himself the attitude of others.[2]

The position Mead takes in his "property" example and the writings of the philosopher John Dewey at around the same time both prefigure the philosopher Ludwig Wittgenstein's later arguments on language.[3] Reversing the position he took in his early writings, Wittgenstein showed in the *Philosophical Investigations* that words are not pointers to objects or situations outside language. Instead, only everyday sentences uttered in social contexts can be said to have meaning, and their meaning derives solely from the social "forms of life" (for example, playing a game; giving an order) of which they are a part. Language simply embodies the shared beliefs and practices of the community of language users.

Once the ideas of Mead and Wittgenstein on the collective nature of language and concepts are understood, the notions of self and self-consciousness can be approached in the same way. According to Mead, consciousness of self is the adoption of the attitude of the generalized other toward oneself. Impelled by the desire to belong, children enter into organizations at first as a kind of social game; the child's self then becomes determined by his relationship with the group to which he belongs. Self-consciousness arises in the process of social experience. The generalized attitude of others toward oneself becomes linked with the sensations of one's body, to produce the feelings of personal existence with which we are familiar.

Although some modern infant researchers seem to imply that individual selves must exist before infants can recognize correspondences between their own behavior and that of others, the developmental psychologist Lev Vygotsky maintained that individual cognition has its origin in transactions with others. He held that the transactions in which infants participate are internalized to create the structure of individual mentation. Children learn social scripts and conventions by participating in them; individual cognition subsequently bears the stamp of its social origins. This would imply, in accordance with Mead, that the child's concept of itself, like its other concepts, arises from interactions with others, rather than existing a priori.

The contemporary social psychologist Rom Harré, speaking in a general rather than a developmental framework, explained more specifically how the experience of having a self derives from the collectively held concept of "person." According to Harré, society's idea of what it means to be a person is an abstract notion, collectively subscribed to, in just the same way as is Mead's concept of property. In having selves, individuals are subscribing to the collective notion of a person, which is particular to their culture. The experience of a self is the result of applying a *theory* to account for the organization of experience. Now, the notion of gravitational fields is a theory used by scientists to account for the movements of physical objects, but when an apple falls on the head of a physicist, he or she does not say, "Ouch! Gravity!" Gravitational fields aren't directly experienced, even by those familiar with the theory. In contrast, in the case of "self," once we have the concept our experiences are directly interpreted as manifestations of "self"—we don't notice that we are applying a theory. To quote Harré,

> when we learn to organize our organically grounded experience as a structured field, and cognitively as a body of beliefs built up of self-predications, we are deploying a concept of "self" that functions like the deep theoretical concepts of the natural sciences, which serve to organize our experience and knowledge, whether or not they have observable referents in the world.
>
> The public-collective concept of "person" is all that is required both to create and to understand this form of structuring. . . .
>
> Consciousness is the product of a complex interweaving of a perceptual-experiential structure and conceptual–theoretical structure, such that experience is attributed to a person. . . . there are both physiological conditions necessary for the existence of consciousness and cultural schemata by which it is structured.[4]

Other thinkers have also viewed the self as a sort of theory. Dennett wrote that we live in a social medium of "words, words, words," which we incorporate and in turn extrude as collections of stories, beliefs, and assertions. He wrote that individuals assign these multiple narratives "a center of narrative gravity" and attach to them a hypothetical "owner of record," which is the self. This account echoes that of William James, who, a century ago, likened thoughts to a herd of cattle, all bearing a common brand. The herd possesses only a potential unity until the herdsman or owner furnishes a real figure to which all the individual beasts belong. Common sense supplies this "owner," the self, an explanation of the apparent unity in the stream of individual thoughts.

The ideas of Mead, Harré, and Dennett regarding subjectivity are fundamentally different from theories of sensory awareness that restrict themselves to the physiology of individual brains. The views of Mead and Harré imply that *only brains in a social field can generate the kind of consciousness that includes "I."* From the perspective of a social constructivist, theories of consciousness that restrict themselves to isolated brain mechanisms can only aspire to explaining subject-less awareness, but not to explaining the *experience of one's self being aware.*[5]

Yet we saw in chapter 1 that people with brain damage can feel as though someone else's subjectivity is taking over their own, or that their own consciousness has been relocated to other bodies. These phenomena indicate that individual human brains have a capacity for assigning subjectivity—both to others and to the self. Can we reconcile the idea that subjectivity is crafted by individual brains with the idea that subjectivity is the product of a social belief system? We can, by realizing that the mind-making organ of the brain operates within a social field. A social field alone is not enough, for autistic children fail to make mind despite being raised in a thoroughly social manner. And a mind-making organ alone is not enough: Society must provide the brain with specific *forms* of self and person, just as it provides the particular language that the brain's language-making organ will take up and reproduce.

To see how the social field and the innate specialization for forming a "self" normally work together, let's consider a situation in which the two were uncoupled and subsequently recoupled, and how the self of a child was affected by these events. Helen Keller was a normally developing child until the age of 19 months, when a serious infectious illness rendered her both blind and deaf. Because of her impairments, participation in the social world was effectively impossible. She continued to be raised at home, but became aggressive and difficult to manage. When she was 6, her parents located a teacher by the name of Anne Sullivan, who came to live in the Keller household and teach the child. The following passages detail the dramatic experiences of both student and teacher at the time Miss Keller stepped into the shared world of language.[6]

On April 3, 1887, a few days before the famous moment at the water pump, Miss Sullivan wrote in her correspondence to a friend, "I spell in her hand everything we do all day long, although she has no idea as yet what the spelling means." On April 5, she began her letter, "I must write you a line this morning because something very important has happened." After some further remarks, she continued:

> We went out to the pumphouse, and I made Helen hold her mug under the spout while I pumped. As the cold water gushed forth, filling the mug, I spelled "w-a-t-e-r" in Helen's free hand. The word coming so close upon the sensation of cold water rushing over her hand seemed to startle her. She dropped the mug and stood as one transfixed. A new light came into her face. She spelled "water" several times. Then she dropped on the ground and asked for its name and pointed to the pump and the trellis, and suddenly turning round she asked for my name. I spelled "Teacher." . . . All the way back to the house she was highly excited.

Several days later, Miss Sullivan wrote of Helen's continuing avidity for words, and added, "We notice that her face grows more expressive each day."

Miss Keller herself wrote in her autobiography that, prior to her education, she was like a ship at sea in a dense fog, "without compass or sounding-line, and had no way of knowing how near the harbor was." On the morning before the experience at the pump, Miss Sullivan had been trying to teach her the word "doll." "I became impatient at her repeated attempts and, seizing the new doll, I dashed it upon the floor. I was keenly delighted when I felt the fragments of the broken doll at my feet. . . . In the still, dark world in which I lived there was no strong sentiment or tenderness."

Following her experience at the pump, which Miss Keller later described as "my soul's sudden awakening," she wrote:

> As we returned to the house every object that I touched seemed to quiver with life. That was because I saw everything with the strange, new sight that had come to me. On entering the door I remembered the doll I had broken. I felt my way to the hearth and picked up the pieces. I tried vainly to put them together. Then my eyes filled with tears; for I realized what I had done, and for the first time I felt repentance and sorrow.

Miss Keller characterized her entry into language as the acquisition of a kind of new sight. Both her own and her teacher's observations surrounding the initiation suggest that more than just the acquisition of an external, tool-using capacity had taken place. A transformation was effected by her entry into a collective world, for it was only through her participation in a collective life that a self became possible. The public nature of this new self is suggested by the expressiveness that emerged, at around the same time, on her face.

The account of the actions with the doll are eloquent: The sensory losses suffered at 19 months of age had shattered a developing self, resulting in an angry and isolated child who nevertheless communicated her situation at a primitive level—by breaking things. When the new self that was created by membership in a language community came into being, it recognized and felt compassion for the old, damaged self as symbolized by the doll. And, finally, this new person was now able to experience the social feelings that bind members of a community with others, such as repentance and love.

During a child's development, faith in shared experience develops from imitation, is first expressed in referential gaze and pointing, and later underpins language. Ultimately, the social field of human beings is created by the ability to take the position of the generalized "other," for, according to the symbolic interactionists, it is only through taking this position that meaning arises for the individual—including the meaning of one's own self. A potential problem with this view might seem to be the implication that individual minds are passive receptacles for static social constructs. Sociologists influenced by the philosopher Charles Peirce understand the self to be a flux of signs, interpreted as "self" by the individual orchestrating their arrangement, and as "person" by those outside to whom the signs are presented. The so-called postmodern view of the individual is that he or she continuously selects from competing semiological codes of self and personhood offered by the culture; in so doing, individuals compose the signs by which they will know themselves and be known by others.[7]

Face-to-face interactions are the small-scale nuts and bolts of social behavior—it is to these that we have related the capacities of the human brain throughout the book. In narratives and performances, individuals actively create themselves as persons, and in collaboration with others, create worlds of meaning. Understanding that people both elaborate social worlds, and enact their places within them, allows communicative episodes to be viewed under the dual aspects that they always simultaneously possess. We now turn from the creation of selves to the creation of social worlds.

Social Brain, Social Mind

Human beings do something strange. We create elaborate, arbitrary worlds and treat them as if they were mundane and inevitable. We cannot see that we do this or how we do this—but we can see that others have done it when their worlds are different from our own. Anthropologists working in remote areas often have to endure being laughed at because they don't know the "obvious." Only a child or a fool would not know that a man must not enter a hut in which one of his male relatives has died, or that it is dangerous to venture out on the night of a new moon. How do such "facts" become so self-evident?

The activity by which people jointly create simple social facts is the subject matter of a field called ethnomethodology. This branch of sociology, originated by the researcher Harold Garfinkel, looks at how commonsense facts—the things that "anyone can see"—are created and perpetuated by people through their talk and actions.[8] It looks, in other words, at how performances and narratives create concepts that then have the character of being objectively true, "really out there in the world" to the participants engaged in their construction. Ethnomethodologists have discovered that the reality of socially constructed categories is underwritten by circular logic: Their factualness is presumed while, at the same time, inherently ambiguous events are brought to bear as evidence of them. This sounds complicated, but it is in fact the pervasive logic of everyday thought. As an example, let's look at a study that showed how teachers found evidence for social types such as "immature child," "independent worker," and "bright student." The sociologist Kenneth Leiter found that various behaviors of children were interpreted by teachers, to themselves, and to each other, as "the document of" or as "pointing to" such underlying categories. The problem was that children's actual behavior was not always consistent with the attributes the teachers had assigned them. Because, if they are real, such attributes must exist independently of variations in behavior, the teachers found ways to account for and dismiss behavior, such as test performance, which did not conform to the attributions they had made. These accountings were carried out by creatively supplying contexts ("she was upset that day") for particular behaviors that otherwise threatened to erode the congruence of the (created) social object. A poor test performance by a "bright student" might have been taken as evidence for her rattled frame of mind, or for the test's being poorly written—but it didn't challenge her assignment to the category "bright student." A villager's going out on the night of a new moon and returning unscathed might be accounted for in the same creative way: He was carrying a special amulet, or a shaman had trod the same path the day before, making it safe. By such methods, underlying "truths" (the student is bright, the new moon is dangerous) are upheld and contrary evidence explained away. Belief in underlying categories is only strengthened, never weakened, by actual events. Ethnomethodologists have called this kind of logic "the documentary method."

The documentary method is usually employed collectively in performances and narratives, so it is a very powerful creator of shared belief. D. Lawrence Wieder, a sociologist who participated in the community he was studying, resided at a halfway house for ex-convicts and learned how a "code" of convict behavior, to which both residents and staff subscribed, was used to account for events and interactions. The code was presented as justification for certain behavior, and members of the community presented themselves to one another as adapting to the code. Wieder's understanding of the code progressed as he participated in the community. What were at first vague principles (ex-convicts don't tell on other ex-convicts) became increasingly elaborated and real for him by the assimilation of actual behaviors as exemplars. Events at the halfway house became, for Wieder, "progressively experienced as more and more complex, elaborate, definite, seeable-in-a-glance"—in short, as direct manifestations of underlying truths. Wieder noted that both he and novice staff members, who were all faced with the common task of understanding halfway house culture, were ultimately able to gear their own actions to those of the residents. Individuals who are born into a culture or who are fully acculturated gear their actions effortlessly to those of the group, whereas novices or outsiders who may be trying to "pass" as members struggle to acquire embedded rules, and thus can only interact successfully with some effort. Native members of a local culture, unlike visiting sociologists or anthropologists, use underlying procedures and concepts tacitly, automatically, and without awareness.

The sociologist Alfred Schutz pointed out that people make two basic assumptions with respect to one another, for the purpose of supposing that a common world transcending their private experience exists. The first is the interchangeability of standpoints. According to this idealization, if I were to take up my partner's place, I would see things as he now does, I would be at the same distance from things that he now is, and so on. The second idealization is the congruency of the system of relevances. This is the assumption that my partner and I subscribe, for all practical purposes, to the same system of relevances in the objects and events with which we are jointly engaged.[9] These assumptions are seen in the actions of babies between 9 months and 1 year of age when they engage their mothers in joint attention to a common object, and when they look to their mothers for evaluations of unusual events, in situations called "social referencing," in order to assign relevance to new and unfamiliar experiences. These two primary assumptions are the results of the infant's "like me" belief. The faith that my world and your world are shared in common creates the following effect: When together we create social objects (for example, categories such as "property" or "immature child"), they become real for both of us. Children, who are new to the practices of co-construction, create shared realities explicitly in pretense ("Let's say this is a store"). Once children have achieved the ability to co-construct reality, the scaffold of pretense falls away, and adult co-construction, which is tacit, supervenes.

Puzzles Resolved

We saw in chapter 5 that Enlightenment thinking saw science as reaching toward an outside, objective truth. In the Enlightenment metaphor, minds and brains were isolated entities that grasped the inanimate world outside. In the present chapter, we have moved to a position in which reality as something "out there" has taken a back seat to reality as something collectively created—like Wittgenstein's replacing the notion of reference in language with the notion of a community of speakers and families of meaning. An alternative to Enlightenment epistemology is called pragmatism. Pragmatism does not deny the existence of an external reality, but pragmatists acknowledge the power of social construction. As a result, they are less sanguine than Enlightenment philosophers about how completely the external world can be made independent from the collective biases of the scientists who study it. In the pragmatist metaphor, mind is defined by its membership in a collective of other minds. The paradigmatic example of Enlightenment neuroscience is the study of vision (the isolated mind that looks out on the world); the paradigmatic example of pragmatist neuroscience is the study of the brain's social responsiveness (minds created by community), the subject of this book.

At first it may seem as though we have left the orderly garden of positivism for the wilderness of social constructionism. But Enlightenment views of the brain had in fact generated a lot of confusion—in other words, the garden was in a bit of a mess. Adopting a social paradigm for brain function helps clear up a set of problems that plagued philosophers and theoretically inclined neuroscientists alike. These sometimes appeared as arguments for the intrinsic dichotomy of the humanities and the natural sciences, and sometimes as "the mind–brain problem."

For example, at the end of the last century, when the natural sciences were enjoying an expansive heyday, the philosopher Wilhelm Dilthey claimed that the human sciences, which included the humanities and social sciences, were independent of the natural sciences.[10] His argument was based on the irreducibility of subjective experience. Using a typically Germanic example, he wrote: "The independent position of such a discipline cannot be contested, so long as no one can claim to make Goethe's life more intelligible by deriving his passions, poetic productivity, and intellectual reflection from the structure of his brain or the properties of his body." The assertion that there is *in principle* a domain outside the explanatory reach of natural science is an affront to the natural science claim that everything in the world is ultimately explainable in physical terms. One can view Dilthey's strong claim for the independent reality of experience as both a reaction to and a mirror of the strong natural science claim for a knowable external reality. The gap created by these polar positions collapses, however, when we extend the natural sciences to include the social functions of the human brain. Communities of socially capable brains, using mechanisms we have described in these pages, produce the collective sphere of thought and language in which we find entities like poetry, reflection, and self-awareness.

The eminent modern biologist Gunther Stent attributed the concept of self to an evolved a priori structure of individual cognition.[11] He wrote that "our brains oblige us" to use everyday concepts such as self, concepts he claimed are insufficient for science. He concluded, therefore, that there could be no scientific understanding of self, or human experience—in principle. Consistent with his Enlightenment epistemology, Stent used the visual system as a model for the brain. What he failed to see was that "self" arises in human communities *because of the brain's built-in apparatus for assigning a locus of subjectivity combined with its adaptation for participating in communally created social objects*. It was not the concept of self that was deficient, preventing a scientific understanding of human experience: Rather, the traditional concept of the brain was deficient. What was needed, but was not available to Stent, was an account of how our brains allow us to attribute subjectivity, and to participate in communities that collectively define self and person.

Philosophers such as Patricia Churchland have thoughtfully considered how conscious awareness might be understood using the language of neuroscience. They have worried, however, about the fate of "meaning" in such an effort. To address the problem, they have conducted "thought experiments," imagining the internal states of isolated automata and puzzling over how these could give rise to meaning.[12] Symbolic interactionists would say that webs of meaning exist not within one individual, but in the expectable behavioral responses of a collectivity, response dispositions to which an individual subscribes at the moment of uttering a sentence. The idea that isolated automata, like little Robinson Crusoes, can be models for human brains that produce meaning is wrong. To model human minds appropriately, researchers are now beginning to situate automata within societies of automata.[13]

In retrospect, the early findings of socially responsive neurons by Gross and Rolls, from squarely within the isolated-brain paradigm, foretold a different, social view of the primate brain. Scientists have begun to describe how brain function underwrites our species' social existence. Although they are still at an early stage in their discoveries, researchers have begun to grapple with how the brain takes in and organizes the flow of social signals that bombard it. Through the processing of social signals, the brain makes descriptions of others' intentions and evaluates the status of their current commitments to mutual action and social objects. Our program in this book has been to approach the brain as an object of empirical investigation, about which hard facts can be discovered. What we want such hard facts to help us understand is how our brains so skillfully and persistently create socially constructed "facts"—among them, ourselves and our social worlds. Because traditional isolated-mind science had no place for socially constructed "facts," they were declared out of bounds. We are now in a position to redraw the boundaries of natural science to include them.

In this chapter, we began to appreciate the workings of everyday logic and how it artfully creates and sustains objects as diverse as the expected behavior of ex-convicts and bright students. The circular logic of the documentary method is very different from the logic of scientific thought, which requires prediction and control in order to be satisfied that understanding has been achieved. Interestingly though, the objects that everyday thinking creates are not always easy to distinguish from those that science discovers—just as the pragmatists would predict. And yet it is not impossible to dissect them from each other.

In the next chapter we take up a topic—emotion—in which socially constructed "facts" have blended together with or replaced scientific facts. The primary aim of the chapter will be to sharpen the distinction between social construction and science in this area. The secondary aim will be to illustrate how difficult it is to keep scientific thought and everyday thought from intermingling. In the end, we will want to take a respectful stance toward the everyday logic that we uncover. Far from regarding everyday thought as science's poor relation, we should maintain a lively appreciation for the rich and compelling worlds it produces. To appreciate these worlds is to appreciate what our brains do best.

8

In Search of Emotion

"Emotion" has no single, defined referent; instead, the word is a pointer to a loose assortment of ideas. On the one hand, it connotes subjective qualities of experience—we call them "feelings." On the other, it connotes expressiveness. Does emotion have any standing as an empirical, scientific entity—or is it just a manner of speaking? A review of current neurobiological theories and findings will lead us to conclude, in agreement with some sociologists, that emotion is a construct of everyday thought and is not to be found in our brains or bodies.

Emotion in the Brain and Body

According to isolated-mind psychologists, emotions are brain states that activate prewired patterns of muscular activity on the face and elsewhere. Paul Ekman, famous for seminal cross-cultural studies of facial expressions, wields considerable influence in the field of emotion. He hints that if we could just look inside the brain, we'd see the tell-tale neural signs of emotion: "Looking from the outside, without access to knowledge of what is occurring in the central nervous system, how can an observer tell when an emotion is present?"[1]

Believing emotions exist somewhere within the brain, psychologists have looked hopefully to neuroscientists to find emotion in the hardware of the brain. And neuroscientists have complied—or tried to. The logical problems they have encountered along the way are instructive. Their failures in fact prove that the isolated-mind concept of emotion must be discarded. Let us trace their efforts.

The preeminent contemporary researcher identified with the study of emotion's neural basis is Joe LeDoux. In his experimental work with rats, LeDoux elegantly demonstrated that a series of nerve signals traveling from auditory centers to the amygdala are responsible for a rat's conditioned response to a sound associated with a noxious stimulus. In addition to his empirical demonstrations, LeDoux made two major theoretical assertions. One held that the larger topic of emotion may be broken down into individual emotions, such as fear, for the purposes of experimental study. The other held that a set of brain structures known as the limbic system, traditionally thought to be the seat of emotional experience, was not defined correctly and needed to be revised.

We turn first to the question of studying individual emotions. Like other workers in the field, LeDoux did not examine the underlying assumption that emotion is a real entity. Assuming that an unseen, underlying entity is responsible for an array of surface phenomena is a hallmark of the documentary method—the everyday logic we looked at in the last chapter. Proceeding with this assumption in place, LeDoux suggested that one might study the neural basis of emotion by breaking it down into basic elements, such as fear, anger, and so forth. In this way, neuroscientists could approach the general subject of emotion by studying one emotion at a time. Separate from these proposals, LeDoux showed in laboratory experiments that pathways in the amygdala were essential for generating a kind of behavior he called "fear conditioning" in the rat. Fear conditioning is produced when a rat learns to associate a tone, for example, with aversive experiences such as electric shock that are experimentally paired with it. Once a rat has learned the association, it will become immobile and undergo characteristic changes of blood pressure and heart rate on hearing the tone. LeDoux's empirical demonstrations regarding the brain basis of fear conditioning were clear examples of scientific logic and method. But he used his scientific results to support documentary reasoning regarding emotion in general.

Having described the amygdala pathway responsible for fear conditioning in the rat, LeDoux considered whether this pathway could be said to be the basis of fear in general. He reviewed many other experimental paradigms said to measure fear but found that they did not all involve this pathway. He remarked that, unlike his own experiments, some of the other fear experiments use active or passive avoidance as behavioral measures, and he noted that the nature of the fear-inducing stimuli varies between laboratories. Based on these considerations, he concluded that the different experiments measure fear to different degrees. "The amygdala has been implicated in most of these tests of fear. However, not all variations of every task have proven to be sensitive to amygdala damage. There are many ways to structure any of these tasks and it is important to ask, for every task and every variation of the task, whether it is truly a measure of fear."[2] In other words, there was a discrepancy between the observed experimental results and the expected results: The amygdala was presumed to be essential for the experience of fear, but the amygdala was not always essential in tasks that apparently involve fear. Under such circumstances, the documentary method calls in creative accounting, as we saw in the last chapter. Rather than question whether the underlying construct is valid, the documentary method accounts for the discrepancy by invoking the particular context—some of the experiments are not pure measures of fear, but involve novelty, or more complex responses, or some other complicating element. Although LeDoux implied that fear exists somehow apart from these diverse paradigms, each of which approaches its measure more or less well, the validity of fear itself was assumed, not demonstrated.

LeDoux assumed that his own fear-conditioning paradigm was the purest measure of the underlying entity, fear. That this assumption is based on flawed logic actually leads to a positive contribution: Although he did not draw this conclusion himself, the obvious implication of his failure is that *fear is a semantic category that does not map onto the various experimental paradigms involving brains and behaviors of rats.* LeDoux could not establish the neural basis of fear, his prototype emotion, *in general*, although he had established a neural basis for "fear conditioning" as specifically defined in his own experiments. His attempt to make a general empirical statement about emotion therefore foundered at its first step. The failure suggested that, like fear, emotion itself would ultimately falter as a meaningful empirical category. In science, failures can be as important as successes, for they cause scientists to question received ideas. The second theoretical assertion that LeDoux made also undermined the concept of emotion, but in a different way.

LeDoux carefully analyzed the limbic system, a historical term for a set of brain structures believed to mediate emotional experience, by testing the evidence and arguments that pointed to the existence of such a system. We will take a moment to summarize LeDoux's thoughtful analysis, for the same arguments that explode the limbic system concept explode the emotion concept as well.[3]

The term *limbic*, meaning edge or bank, was coined by the anatomist Paul Broca to designate a set of structures on the inner wall of the cerebral hemispheres ("le grand lobe limbique"). Although it was at first assumed that limbic structures served olfactory functions,

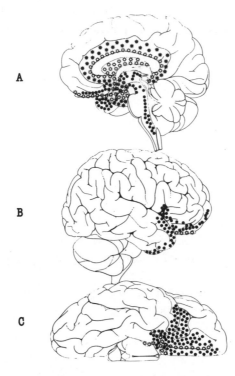

Figure 8.1.   Areas of the brain often included in or associated with the limbic system. (Adapted from Macchi, 1989. Courtesy G. Macchi.) (*Top*) Medial view—that is, from inside a hemisphere. Front of the brain is to the left. (*Middle*) Lateral view—that is, from outside a hemisphere. Front of the brain is to the right. (*Bottom*) Ventral view—that is, from below a hemisphere. Front of the brain is to the right.

because of their association with olfactory structures, another anatomist by the name of James Papez proposed that some of these structures were part of a neural circuit subserving emotional experience. A number of scientists suggested candidates for inclusion in this circuit, including the cingulate gyrus, hippocampal formation, mammillary bodies, anterior thalamus, hypothalamus, orbitofrontal cortex, insula, anterior temporal cortex, amygdala, and dorsomedial nucleus of the thalamus. The psychiatrist Paul MacLean, picking up the term first used by Broca, designated these structures as "the limbic system."[4] A fairly inclusive list of limbic structures is depicted in Figure 8.1.

LeDoux wrote that the idea of a limbic system is basically an idea about the functional localization of emotion in the brain and outlined the history of the concept as follows. Although the psychologist William James had held that no special emotional centers exist in the brain, later authors named candidate brain structures. The physiologist Walter Cannon believed certain pathways served emotional *expression*, whereas others served subjective emotional *experience*. Papez elaborated on Cannon's account, by describing a route for adding what he called "emotional coloration" to cognition. MacLean packaged the ideas of both Cannon and Papez into a functional system, which he held to be primarily dedicated to emotional experience and expression. It is this system that is labeled the limbic system.

LeDoux showed that there were four basic assumptions embedded in MacLean's concept. He examined each of them in turn. One was that anatomical criteria could be used for assigning brain structures to the limbic system. In fact, no consistent set of criteria coincide with experimental findings on involvement with emotion. A second assumption is that brain regions that are members of the limbic system are all involved in visceral regulation (that is, they control smooth muscle structures such as blood vessels and the gastrointestinal tract): This too does not hold up. A third assumption is that visceral changes are the basis of emotion. LeDoux argued that it is unlikely that the viscera can respond with enough speed or specificity to be the bodily basis of different emotions. Finally, LeDoux showed that emotion is not the only, or even the main, function of so-called limbic structures.

What LeDoux showed, in effect, is that the so-called limbic system is a reification of emotion in the brain. LeDoux himself, however, was very clear in asserting that the brain must in fact contain an emotional system: He did not attack the assumption that underlay the reification, but simply sought to revise the criteria for qualifying a brain structure as involved in emotion. Having extensively reviewed findings from a large number of experiments using stimulation, lesions, fear conditioning, avoidance learning, and experimental anxiety, he selected the amygdala and orbital frontal cortex, and rejected the hippocampus, as proposed members of an emotional circuit. He wrote, "some other limbic areas . . . appear to contribute to emotion, but their contributions remain less clear." [5] Was LeDoux struggling to describe the clothes on a naked emperor?

What is unclear is the emotion concept itself. Being unclear, the concept inevitably makes analysis of the so-called emotional functions of various brain areas unclear. To begin with, how does the investigator know when he or she sees an emotion? LeDoux included attacking, fighting, fleeing, and feeding in a list of "species-typical emotional behaviors." He listed typical signs of fear in the laboratory rat as "freezing" (becoming immobile), raising of the hair, and increases in blood pressure and heart rate. How do these relate to emotion? When experimenters stimulate brain areas classically designated "limbic" in experimental animals, they see such species-typical behaviors, which *appear to indicate that the animal is having an intense subjective experience.* That is, experimenters make an imaginative move, constructing the presence of an unseen entity called emotion, taking as evidence for its presence such elements as raised hair and increased heart rate. This also amounts to a reification, for a neural substrate of emotion seems to be confirmed at exactly the same time. The fact that speakers of the English language generally agree on how to use the word "emotion" does not automatically mean that emotion must exist in the natural world as a definable set of physical processes, however.

In fact, we use the term emotion to speak about an individual's subjective experience as opposed to his or her actions or other objective states of the world. Although the content is not critical to our idea of emotion—for the actual content of the experience may be anything from hunger to panic to remorse—a certain kind of intensity seems to be connoted by the word. In short, there is a semantic kinship between the concept of emotion and the general idea of intense subjective experience. This kinship brings emotion smack into a thorny philosophical realm designated by the term *qualia*. Qualia refers to the qualities of subjective experience—for example, how pain *feels* or what it is like to see the color red—as opposed to the brain states that painful stimuli or red objects might cause, states that could be measured by an outside observer but not felt. Indeed, the apparent kinship between emotion and intense subjective experience implies that emotion is like qualia— only more so! Unless emotion is reduced to physical behavior, the problem of qualia must be dealt with. But if neuroscientists can be said to have one healthy, justified "emotion," it is fear of qualia. That is because proposals for the relationship between qualia and brain states have a long, convoluted, and entirely unsatisfactory history.

Dennett has suggested a way out of the problems that qualia poses for researchers, and his solution points the way to how emotion should be dealt with as well. He argues that, over long periods of time, biases have gotten built into our nervous systems because of selection pressure. To take a simple example, the sight of a snake tends to produce the physical ingredients of readiness to flee, such as the release of adrenaline; it also produces more complex, inborn associations relating to violence and damage. Culturally learned associations are triggered as well. Dennett argues that the subjective qualities of the sight of a snake or the color pink, or the sound of a piece of music, are none other than the bundle of action tendencies, both inborn and learned, that each of these calls forth.[6]

Imagine a continuum of subjective experience, which ranges from your experience of an abstract idea, your experience of a word, or your experience of a color on one end, to your experience of the approach of someone who is about to tear you limb from limb on the other. On the "cool" end of the spectrum, the experiences elicit complex associations and tendencies to respond, but these only gently nudge us toward action. That is what qualia are, the sum of associated action dispositions. Why are emotions "emotional"? They are emotional because, at the "hot" end of the spectrum of subjective experience, the information that is being processed is tightly coupled with physical states of response, unlike the looser coupling at the cool end. That is, our brains are made so that the features of a looming rival are processed in areas directly responsible for generating adrenaline and other components of flight. When brain regions that recruit body responses act in concert, action becomes imminent. The greater the coherence and imminence of bodily response, the greater the intensity of feeling. But "feeling" is not something separate from and additional to the bodily response—it is simply our way of talking about the bodily response.

Now we are in a position to understand why the myth of the limbic system has had such a hold on the neuroscientific imagination. There are certain areas in the brain that receive a confluence of sensory input in a variety of modalities and in turn are directly coupled to other regions that cause changes in bodily states, such as heart rate, pupil size, hormone levels, and muscle activity. The areas that have been most universally agreed to belong to "the limbic system" are those that possess this input–output pattern to the greatest degree. When animals or humans undergo electrical stimulation of these brain regions, they give every indication that they are registering a situation imperatively linked to physical action—be it running away, assuming a defensive fighting posture, or becoming aroused for sexual activity. "Limbic" brain regions, in other words, are where sensory activity is most tightly linked to changes in the body. Strong action tendencies linked with their eliciting sensory contexts—such as the tears that well in our eyes when parting with a loved one, the sinking sensation in our stomachs when we imagine a dreaded confrontation, or the desire to dance a jig when disaster is averted—these are the experiences we call "emotions." There is no sharp distinction between the concept of emotion and that of subjective experience in general, just the tendency to use the term emotion when body states are more mobilized.[7]

The neurologist and neuroscientist Antonio Damasio has argued eloquently for the role of the body in states of subjective feeling, describing how our brains register changes in body states of all kinds, be they subtle changes in blood flow or overt muscle activity.[8] Although he retains the language of emotion and feeling, many of his statements reveal the centrality of action dispositions in his theory. Because Damasio does not question the assumption that emotion is a valid category, however, he is forced to make a distinction between body states that are emotional and those that are not—otherwise, emotion would have no standing as a category separate from the body's dispositions to act. To make this distinction, Damasio separates what he calls "background feelings" from emotional states, saying that the former are more restricted in range and that they correspond to nonemotional body states, a somewhat circular definition. We may readily accede to the idea that emotional states are somehow different from nonemotional states. But is this because there *is* a discrete, objective dividing line between body states in one and not the other condition that we can demonstrate? Or is it because we tacitly but mistakenly insist, in advance, that there are such things as emotions that *must* in some way be different from other subjective experiences?

We have knocked down a house of cards, in which each card represented a set of ideas underpinning still other ideas. Following Dennett, if we equate subjective experience with action tendencies, we cannot say emotion is a *qualitatively distinct* kind of subjective experience, only that action tendencies may be more or less acute. And without emotion, there is no need for "brain circuitry underlying emotion." In fact, the notion that there is a brain basis of emotion had been seriously weakened by LeDoux's deconstruction of the limbic system concept, together with the logical flaws in his search for the emotion "fear" in an experimental setting. We now turn to another aspect of the emotion concept, expression.

Emotion as Communication

What about facial expressions? Aren't they signs of inner emotion? In our answer we will keep in mind that the emotion construct is problematic to the extent that its semantics cluster around minds as isolated entities with "feelings" that are independent of physical dispositions to act. Our trouble in understanding facial expressions emerges when we link them with emotion as an isolated, inner state. As we move away from biology and adopt the language of sociology, however, emotions begin to be conceived as essentially interpersonal communicative acts. In this section we will see how expressive behaviors can be considered in the context of mutually regulating systems of behavior, rather than in the context of inner states.

Two basic positions regarding facial expressions may be expressed in extreme form as follows. According to the first, inner states are "readouts" onto the face. This position ties facial expressions to private, inner emotions. The private becomes public through facial expressions: Emotional faces are "evolved, biologically based, involuntary signs of felt emotion."[9] Facial expressions generated during everyday social interactions between people, according to this view, are distortions of the "pure" emotional faces, which socialization has modified in accordance with cultural rules. Therefore, facial expressions seen in everyday life consist of "pure" emotions, "blends" of pure emotions, or underlying pure emotions modified by display rules. The psychologist Alan Fridlund has suggested that the appeal of such an account is romantic, for it refers implicitly to "an 'authentic self', independent of social relations, manifest in heartfelt emotion erupting on the face."[10]

At the other extreme is the view that facial signals are primarily communicative, and therefore sensitive to the outside context rather than the inside milieu. This account holds that facial displays serve solely to regulate social interactions. And indeed, we know that social contexts may determine the communicative displays that animals produce. For example, when roosters are exposed to models of overhead predators, they produce more alarm calls when another chicken is present than when they are alone. The response is fairly specific: When roosters are in the presence of their own mates, they give many more alarm calls in response to a predator than when they are in the presence of familiar females belonging to different fowl species.

Likewise, human facial expressions are to some degree dependent on social context. The psychologists Robert Kraut and Robert Johnston showed that bowlers who had made a strike did not smile when their backs were toward their audiences, but did so when they turned to face their audiences. The fact that people make facial expressions when they are alone has to be interpreted in light of the fact that those who are temporarily alone are often imagining the presence of others. In fact, it has been shown that the more someone imagines others to be present, the greater the tendency to smile, irrespective of how happy the person rates himself to be. Stories communicated in face-to-face situations produce much larger facial expressions in listeners than do stories communicated, for example, by telephone. All the foregoing support the notion that facial expressions are used as signals to others, and that their production therefore depends on social context.[11]

The two positions—that expressions are readouts of inner states and that they are context-sensitive social signals—only appear to be mutually exclusive when thus artificially polarized around the concepts of "inner" and "outer." Some scientists have taken a more intermediate position. For example, Paul Ekman and his colleague Wallace Friesen suggested that "emotional" facial expressions are but one class of expressions, which are found interspersed with other classes— namely, paralinguistic and symbolic facial gestures. Others have gone further, suggesting that the classical "emotional" expressions are just as communicative and interactive as paralinguistic displays.[12] In chapter 6 we saw that both "raw" expressions of "emotion" and highly culturally constrained facial movements occurring in conversation belong to evolved systems for the mutual regulation of behavior. Most researchers would agree that all facial gestures are sensitive to social context. And all facial gestures, just like other bodily responses, are actions. By now we have seen that action or action disposition is the scientific version of the everyday term *feeling*. So we need not keep the idea of an "inner state," which gives rise to facial expressions, for an expression, in this sense, *is* a feeling—and it is also a context-sensitive signal.

A corollary of the isolated-mind view of emotion is that there is a set of "basic" emotions. There is no agreement on exactly which emotions are to be included, however; thus, one proposed set of basic emotions is expectancy, fear, rage, and panic, another is happiness, surprise, fear, sadness, anger, and disgust, and so on. A review of proposed sets of basic emotions reveals there is no consensus either on the number of basic emotions, or on what they are. Because of this disarray, and for theoretical reasons, the psychologists Andrew Ortony and Terence Turner have questioned whether the concept of a "basic emotion" can be valid at all. They conclude that there are no criteria we can use to qualify an emotion as "basic."[13] The considerations offered here against the idea of an isolated-mind emotion, together with the proposal that we think in terms of evolved layers of neural equipment for communication, with newer mechanisms layered on older ones, suggest that trying to get at anything "basic" will probably not be fruitful theoretically. LeDoux's efforts with fear suggest it is not fruitful empirically.

In line with the concept of "basic" emotions, it is often supposed that certain highly stereotyped facial expressions are documents of such discrete, inner emotional states. Psychologists Nancy Etcoff and John Magee converted pictures of faces with prototypical expressions—such as sadness, anger, and surprise—into line drawings using computer graphics. They generated a series of faces such that each prototypical expression was gradually transformed into another expression. For example, over a series of 11 drawings, an angry face changed little by little to become a sad face. In another series, a happy face gradually became a surprised face, and so on. The amount of physical difference between each line drawing and the next in the series was the same. When subjects were asked to look at the faces and identify the expressions, however, their perceptions changed abruptly midway through each series rather than gradually throughout the series. When subjects looked at a series of faces that changed gradually from expressions of anger to expressions of fear, for example, they did not label the faces in the middle of the series as containing a mixture of anger and fear, but saw them as either angry or fearful.[14]

These interesting results do not tell us that people "have" discrete emotions inside that produce prototypical facial expressions outside or that cause them to register others' expressions in a discrete rather than a continuous manner. What they do tell us is that the signal values of expressive faces fall into discrete categories. That is, all facial expressions that generally resemble "anger" have but a single response value for the observer; when the expression shifts toward fear, the response value for the observer immediately becomes qualitatively different. One can imagine that, for our ancestors, a quick and appropriate distinction between another's threatening versus fearful signals was imperative. Perhaps an underlying, evolutionarily ancient, perceptual machinery for such a distinction is revealed in the Etcoff and Magee experiment. Such perceptual mechanisms may have formed the foundation for the way we currently perceive subtle combinations of facial movements during speech, the movements that tell us we are being kidded, that our interlocutor is ready to end the conversation, or that we are about to be told something particularly worthy of attention. In any case, how facial expressions are perceived does not speak either for or against the assumption that there are basic, "inner" emotions.

Sociological Views of Emotion

Neurobiologists' views of emotion tend to minimize the role of social factors, emphasizing instead an underlying, socially isolated biological entity. When we compare their views to those of sociologists, we find that we can divide sociologists into two groups, roughly speaking. The first group differs from the neurobiologists only in the extent to which they emphasize social factors. These sociologists do not question the empirical reality of emotion. Their task is to explain how social factors influence underlying biological entities to produce emotional experience.

For example, Theodore Kemper argues that certain basic "primary" patterns of autonomic activity are experienced in ways conditioned by socialization to produce a myriad of possible emotions that he calls "secondary." Arlie Hochschild writes that individuals evoke and suppress emotions according to the rules of their culture, thus following "feeling rules." To do this, they must manage their own thoughts, their expressions, and even "physical symptoms of emotion." If shaking is not in accordance with the feeling rules for a situation, one attempts to suppress shaking. These examples reveal implicit acceptance of an asocial, biological kernel at the heart of socialized emotion.[15]

A second, more radical, group of sociologists believes that emotions are cultural elements through and through. Instead of inferring the presence of emotion as a prior reality, these sociologists examine how emotions are made real and accepted as real by participants in social interactions. Robert Perinbanayagam writes that "emotions . . . are vocabularies used in the definition of situations" and that "the body's impulses are transformed into concrete and separate signs." Examining the logical grammar of emotion concepts, Jeff Coulter states that "emotions are not logically separable from their conventionalized modes of public display and their logically possible objects of orientation." The same writers, however, appear to have some residual discomfort with the physical phenomena of emotion. Perinbanayagam endorses Hochschild's view that bodily sensations "cooperate" with symbolic constructions; Coulter proposes that physiological substrates be seen as enabling or facilitating, but not causing, emotion. He further suggests that emotion might be studied on separate levels, biological and sociological.[16]

I think it is possible to be thoroughly sociological about emotions. To do so depends on seeing the body and its changes as essentially public and communicative. Actions mediated by the autonomic nervous system are elements from a prehistoric social rhetoric of the body that still persists in us. Sudden urination is a signal; so are blushing and perspiring. Evocative signs, such as pallor, urine, or trembling, are both more primitive and less historically evanescent than, for example, an orchestrated swoon in a cushioned salon or an upraised middle finger in a traffic intersection. Nevertheless, what the ancient and modern physical demonstrations have in common is that they came into being in historical situations that were and are fundamentally social. It is hardly surprising, furthermore, to find new and old signaling systems operating at the same time, either in harmony or dissonance with one another, to produce whole social gestures. These whole gestures must then be interpreted by others and by oneself.

Evolved Systems for the Mutual Regulation of Behavior

It is interesting that the psychologists Carroll Izard and O. Maurice Haynes describe a proposed basic emotion, contempt, in a way that implicitly involves mutual behavioral regulation:

> The prototypical contempt expression is the human sneer, the homologue of the infrahuman snarl. The head tilt and rotation of contempt may have evolved from a movement that makes the canine more visible in the snarl. The eyes rotated in the same direction as the exposed canine keeps the target animal in the field of vision so its reaction to the expression can be observed.[17]

This description is rife with reciprocal signaling. The snarl is a sign to the outside, or "other": Simultaneously, the attitude of the other, as signaled by its visible response, is registered as a sign back to the gesturer.

By now it should be clear that emotion cannot be defined with reference to the mind or body of only one animal or person. Attempts to do so have relied on the circular reasoning that is characteristic of everyday, but not scientific, thought. If we are to retain the word emotion at all, we should think of it in the context of evolved systems for the mutual regulation of behavior, often involving bodily changes that act as signals. The traditional emotion concept, with its connotations of isolated feelings and expression, should be replaced by the notion of a communicative loop of signaling and response. The sender of a signal—for example, a facial expression of knitted brows and bared teeth—triggers a complementary state in the receiver that causes, through evolutionarily inscribed pathways, a state of "being threatened." This state consists of complex bodily dispositions to act, such as release of fight-or-flight hormones, changes in blood pressure, cringing, and so on. "Anger" and "submissive fear" are two complementary behaviors, one of which triggers the other—and the significance of the threatening expression is given by the bodily changes it evokes in its recipient. In the tradition of symbolic interactionism, introduced in chapter 7, we can say that the meaning of the threatening facial display comes into being through what it calls forth in the other. To the extent that the recipient's reaction is assigned by society in general to the triggering facial threat, the threat "means threat." Otherwise, the threat is an action pattern that serves as a releaser of complementary actions, and nothing more.

Even in such a relational framework, we must not fall prey to the idea that there is some overarching entity, emotion, that underlies all the various responses of organisms to their environments. Each response is specific: Each involves a specific context and most likely a unique set of brain pathways that produce action. It is important to study each situation in its own terms and not unify them prematurely just to give ourselves the gratification of wielding an all-encompassing concept.

What about the development of social signaling and experience in children? The implication of the relational view is that a young child's gesture has no meaning in itself and does not refer to or reflect an inner state. Let us use proud, expansive behavior as an example. The infant pulls itself to a standing position, holds on, and bobs up and down, bright-eyed. In the affective matching routines so well described by the psychologist Daniel Stern, the nearby parent might say with exaggerated joyful intonation, "He-e-ey! He-e-ey! Big *girl*! Standing *up!*" accompanying these sounds with lifted eyebrows and a smile.[18] It is this response, given back to the infant, which *becomes* her expansive subjective experience. The bobbing display does not "mean" the infant is proud: Instead, it is a display eliciting expansive parental behavior, which supplies for the infant the meaning of her movements. Later, the eliciting movements can be practiced with the memory of an audience, still retaining their essentially public character, even when the child is alone. Evolution has supplied infants with various eliciting behaviors, and adult caregivers with responsive behaviors (in the case of some adults, richly responsive, and in the case of others, unfortunately, meagerly so). The subjective meanings of their own experiences are given to human babies from the outside. They do not reside within the behaviors themselves.

Emotion in Everyday Talk

Despite unwitting symbolic interactionist descriptions such as that of contempt cited previously, the predominant use of the term "emotion" by neuroscientists and many psychologists draws on isolated-mind thinking. By now, we have seen that "emotion" cannot be located in any actual neural system or body state. For scientists, the elimination of such everyday, nonscientific concepts and their replacement by empirically testable concepts is desirable. Scientists are more likely to get at the truth of how the brain works when they are not impeded by ideas imported from everyday culture. If the arguments I have made here are accepted, scientists may come to eliminate the term "emotion" from their discussions, just as many have already eliminated the term "limbic system."

But in the arena of everyday human affairs, which is a different world, emotion is very real. It is subscribed to in narratives and performances, and "revealed" by the documentary method. It is part of our informal, commonsense model of ourselves. Concepts like emotion inform and shape our very consciousness.[19] What the network of millions of everyday conversations does—and I will illustrate this in detail in the next chapter using psychoanalysis as a variant of everyday conversation—is to shape individual consciousness through the impress of social meaning onto experience. For example, in the case of emotion, it is transparently clear to us (including the neuroscientists among us, who are members of the culture at large before they are neuroscientists) that we are "having an emotion" when certain changes come over us in certain situations. As much as I may have dismantled the concept of emotion in this chapter, emotion still holds sway over me and my readers. It has held sway, and will continue to hold sway, as a way of experiencing myself. It would only cease to do so in a hypothetical society in which everyone talked about it and thought about it differently.

In the next chapter, which deals with psychoanalysis, we turn our attention to the active weaving of experience by a specialized "theoretical" system akin to the theoretical system of everyday life. By putting these two chapters together, I hope to complete a circle between neuroscience and the social construction of mind. In the present chapter I have shown that we cannot use everyday "commonsense" concepts—such as emotion—to explain brain processes. But we can and should use brain processes, the processes I have described in this book that keep us in constant contact through conversation, to explain the existence of everyday concepts. Moreover, just as millions of mundane conversations produce widely shared convictions about the "obvious," specialized conversation produces convictions in its participants as well. And so we turn to psychoanalysis.

9

$\mathcal{P}$sychoanalytic $\mathcal{P}$erformances and $\mathcal{N}$arratives

Psychoanalysis and the Isolated Mind

We saw in chapters 7 and 8 that everyday thought takes surface events as evidence for the reality of other, invisible things. We saw how teachers take the behavior of their pupils as evidence for underlying types such as "independent worker" or "immature child" and researchers take heart rate changes in rats as evidence for "emotion" using the documentary method. Just as external events can be taken as evidence for other, unseen entities, an individual's actions, gestures, and speech can be taken as evidence not only for a self, but for whatever underlying mental categories the culture provides. Sigmund Freud invented a detailed and imaginative network of such categories, a network that became the basis of psychoanalysis. As we take a closer look at this fascinating system, we will see that its logic is much like that of everyday thought. Moreover, just as in everyday interaction, selves are created in psychoanalysis through narratives and performances.

Psychoanalysis is not a science. To see why, let's compare it to astronomy. One of the hard-won triumphs of physical science was the discovery of laws governing planetary movements: Equipped with such knowledge and a telescope, astronomers since Copernicus have been able to deliver commentaries on celestial activities that were impossible in the pre-Copernican era. In apparent similarity, Freud and his followers were able to comment on people's actions and utterances in ways that were completely new. They believed that he also had discovered something previously unknown—namely, a human mental apparatus governed by the unconscious, which operates according to certain laws. But to be scientific, theories must strive to make correct predictions or demonstrate control of the phenomena under study. Astronomers can and do predict the positions of heavenly bodies, but psychoanalysts do not make efforts to test predictions regarding either mental states or behavior. Furthermore, the validation of a theory must not depend on the assent of the object being studied. An analyst may offer the interpretation that a dream is the disguised expression of a particular wish, the dreamer may agree, and the issue is considered settled; this is very different from the way we seek proof that a planet has a certain trajectory, for we don't use the planet's opinion as evidence![1] Critics of Freud have said correctly that his theories are not scientific, but scientistic—that is, they have only the trappings of empirical science.

The natural science attitude toward reality and knowledge infused Freud's conceptualizations of his activity with his patients. In this framework, observers may be in more or less privileged positions with respect to an observer-independent reality. For example, scientists and doctors are supposed to be relatively more privileged than laypersons and patients. In psychoanalysis, the unequal access to truth takes two forms. First, psychoanalytic patients have often been assigned the unprivileged position of the one who distorts some reality about the world, whereas the analyst or therapist has the more comfortable position of being the one who is in touch with reality and, if all goes well, the one who will help the patient overcome his epistemological limitations.

The inequality of privilege also shows itself in this second way: One participant is ignorant of some set of facts about his or her unconscious processes, and the other either knows, or is in charge of conducting the investigation of these facts. Freud likened psychoanalysis to surgery, in which the doctor maintains an objective distance from the flesh on which she or he is operating. The progressive revelations about the patient's intrapsychic reality, handed to the patient by the analyst, have been termed "insights." Insight was classically held to be curative. Words and phrases that characterize this classical view of the psychoanalytic situation are, for example, "reconstruction," "discovery," "historical truth," "veridical interpretation." All refer confidently to a reality that is uncovered.

A subsequent development in psychoanalysis was the replacement of quasi-biological notions such as drives and the unconscious with the terminology of texts or narratives. We will briefly examine the contributions of two proponents of the narrative view of psychoanalysis, Donald Spence and Roy Schafer.[2] It will become apparent that the trouble with their approach is that it emphasizes isolated text making.

Whereas Freud concentrated on Robinson Crusoe's mental apparatus, the narrativists concentrate on Crusoe's diary.

Spence's formulation is a mixture of natural science and narrativist ideas. He rightly perceives the analytic situation, and beyond it the conversations of clinicians, to be a sea of interacting texts. He poses himself the problem of securing special status for a single truth in this threatened flood of multiple, jointly determined meanings. To solve it, he erects a dike composed of several elements—namely, the privileging of one narrative over others, the retention of a distinction between information (historical truth) and storytelling (narrative truth), and a view of language as a medium that obscures true, raw experience. Here is Spence:

> An outside reader, that is, a psychoanalyst with normative competence, hears a session without the background assumptions in the treating analyst at the time of the session. Thus the transcribed session multiplies into a universe of different "texts," the number of texts corresponding to the number of persons reading. Some way must be found to provide the necessary context in order to eliminate these spurious texts. We will call this step the naturalization of the transcript. . . .
>
>   Once it becomes clear that the analyst is engaged in constructive listening much of the time, then the role of background theory changes from that of an abstract superstructure, to be distinguished from the so-called "clinical" theory, to an active presence in the clinical encounter which specifically affects what he hears and how he chooses to respond. Once we give up the idea of evenly-hovering attention, then it becomes all the more important to know what assumptions the analyst is making to supplement the patient's associations.

In other words, "spurious" texts need to be cleared away from the one true text, and the text-making activity that structures the analyst's listening needs to be taken into account—not because it is an inevitable part of the clinical situation, but because it contaminates by interpenetration the "true" material emerging from the patient's pristine subjectivity. In effect, Spence hopes to grasp the isolated subjectivity of the patient by holding at bay all the forces tending to bring it into the sphere of social construction. His task looks to be difficult.

Schafer, on the other hand, writes: "Psychoanalysis is conducted as a dialogue. . . . A life is re-authored as it is co-authored."[3] Although this sounds promising, in Schafer's account the lion's share of the co-authoring belongs to the analyst. For one thing, the patient does not have a very significant role in structuring the analytic narrative: Schafer describes at length how a patient's response to an interpretation can be taken by the analyst in such a way as to confirm the analyst's existing theories, thus casting doubt on the "privilege" presumably enjoyed by the patient in the analytic dialogue. Following these fairly extensive illustrations, he only briefly notes that, in principle, an analyst should be prepared to revise his interpretive conjectures in response to a patient's rejoinder. For another thing, there is no account of how the patient, for his part, arrives at a sense of conviction about the narratives that the analyst is weaving. By leaving out the patient's participation as an experiencing *subject*, Schafer can assert, and does assert, that applied psychoanalysis, which is the use of analytic theories to elaborate on texts such as novels or works of art, is no different than the analysis that takes place in the consulting room. In both cases, according to Schafer, indeterminate texts are "recovered" by the interpretive work of the reader (in the case of a poem) or the analyst (in the case of a patient). That a poem does not revise *its view of itself* as a result of dialogic interaction with a reader shows us that Schafer's account limits itself to one textmaker, the analyst. Schafer's psychoanalysis is not a conversation between two persons. Thus, the narrativist school remains an isolated-mind psychology, in which mental entities, analogous to "deep structures," are objects of knowledge through hermeneutical analysis.

We now turn to precursors of the view of psychoanalysis as a specialized conversation. Many decades ago, psychoanalysts proposed that psychoanalysis is a "two-body" endeavor. The history and vicissitudes of two-body thinking in psychoanalysis began with workers such as Sandor Ferenczi, who experimented with mutual analysis, W. Ronald D. Fairbairn, and Harry Stack Sullivan. Sullivan chose to work and write outside the classical Freudian paradigm. But both Fairbairn and Sullivan emphasized the essential role of interpersonal relations in forming the self.[4]

According to relational models, events in a psychoanalysis are not determined by something solely within the patient that is allowed to emerge and become explicated against the background of the analyst's unexpressive neutrality; instead, events arise as a result of interactions between the patient and the analyst. The analyst's own structuring activity, even if that activity takes the form of silence, is used by the patient in creating his experience of the analysis. What relational theories have in common with the classical model is acknowledgment of the importance of the patient's past in structuring his experience of the present. The classical model, however, concerns itself with the historical development of the patient's drives; the relational model concerns itself with the historical development of the patient's relationships. Relational thinking among psychoanalysts has shown itself in various forms in the object relations school, and most recently in the writing of Robert Stolorow, George Atwood, and Bernard Brandchaft on intersubjectivity.

Intersubjectivity theory explicitly attempts to rid psychoanalysis of remaining vestiges of the isolated-mind paradigm. Stolorow and Atwood discussed and reconstrued the classical topics of psychoanalysis in relational terms. For example, the Freudian concept of drives as biological forces that originate within the isolated mind and organism, and that reside in repressed form in the unconscious, was replaced with formulations that take into account emotional states. According to these authors, to the extent that the child's emotional state fails to elicit attuned responses from caregivers, it is walled off. Such defensively sequestered states, and not repressed instinctual drives, are the basis for the dynamic unconscious. Regarding the analytic dialogue, Stolorow and Atwood wrote: "Since the patient's experience of the therapeutic relationship is codetermined by the organizing activities of both participants in the therapeutic dialogue, the domain of analytic investigation must encompass the entire intersubjective field created by the interplay between the subjective worlds of patient and therapist."[5]

These writers' efforts to expunge the isolated mind were incomplete, however. Terms such as "investigate" are similar to the empirically oriented language Freud and his followers used to describe their approach to uncovering elements of the isolated mental apparatus. Indeed, Stolorow and Atwood acknowledged that their approach was "perspectivalist," in that it "assumes the existence of the patient's psychic reality but claims only to be able to approximate this reality from within the particularized scope of the analyst's own perspective." The alternative to their position, they stated, would be a radical relativism that denies the existence of a psychic reality that can be known.

To this I would reply that there is not a knowable psychic reality outside the ongoing conversation. Both intersubjective perspectivalism and radical relativism are problematic, for they imply that forms of subjective experience are empirical objects, the manifestations of underlying psychic realities.

Psychoanalysis as Conversation

Psychoanalysis is a specialized culture whose central narratives concern subjective experience. What, though, is an experiencing subject? As we saw in chapter 7, when we refer in everyday language to "myself," we are using the concept of person in its first-person form. Self-experience comes about through our participation in a network of acts and stories derived from the local culture—in other words, selves are the sum of acts and stories that depict self. Therefore, when a psychoanalyst confronts an experiencing subject, he or she is face to face, as the hermeneuticists recognized, with performances and narratives. Despite language that refers to a self somehow beneath or behind the public performances that create and depict it, psychoanalysis operates at the interactive surface. It produces its effects through culturally specific performances and narratives—just as everyday culture does.

Psychoanalytic practitioners acculturate patients and each other in standard ways. First, there are narratives. Without necessarily being aware of it, the analyst throws out a conceptual net, like the convicts in the halfway house, to the patient-novice. This net takes bits of the patient's subjective experience and offers them back as evidence of abstract forms, structures, motivations. These forms may be drives, object relations, or self-objects, depending on the analyst's background. The patient acquires parts, sometimes only fragments, of the net and, in doing so, is psychoanalytically acculturated. In this process, he or she comes to reinterpret his or her experience (or to newly interpret previously uninterpreted experiences) in the light of a new system. But reinterpretation does not quite capture the immediacy, the seeable-in-a-glance nature of the patient's new convictions. The patient's very self appears to him or her in a new light. Subjective experiences now have new meanings. By adopting the new conceptual system, and making it his or her own, the patient creates a new experience of him- or herself.[6]

Second, psychoanalytic reality is mediated by here-and-now performances, streams of signs that may be linguistic or not. Conversation in the consulting room may take place in the extended sense described by Harré as "any flow of interactions brought about through the use of a public semiotic system."[7] In addition to narrative, psychoanalysis has its own semiotic systems, often created de novo by particular analyst–patient pairs. These involve such things as the schedule, the couch, how much silence there is, and other aspects of the relationship normally referred to as "the frame." Because the analyst is trained to notice the performative aspects of the analytic conversation, both verbal and nonverbal, he or she assumes responsibility for making these elements explicit. With a degree of recursiveness that would be unusual in nonanalytic conversations, performative elements may themselves become topics of discussion.

As in other social settings, psychoanalytic participants act jointly. The analyst must be able to enter into the narratives and performances launched at him or her by the patient, picking them up and weaving them together with his or her own system of behavior. The richness and flexibility of the analyst's narratives, and his or her ability *jointly with the patient* to create plausible links between them and bits of the patient's experience and behavior, together constitute the analyst's necessary equipment. The patient must be able to elaborate new narratives and reinterpret his or her experiences: In old-fashioned terminology these were called "capacity for insight" and "psychological mindedness." When all these ingredients are present, a setting is created in which a new experience of self—which is to say, a new self—can come into being. The ingredients of this new self lie in the structure of the mini-society formed by the particular pair, through the narrative networks and enactments in which they jointly and unpredictably engage.

Psychoanalysts also acculturate each other in training analyses, supervision, and case conferences. In the latter two settings, an analyst demonstrates to others how he or she understood a patient's "material." What the analyst relates is, in fact, the conversation; and this relating becomes the starting point for yet another conversation, a conversation between clinicians. Over and over again, psychoanalytic culture replicates itself in narratives concerning subjective experience. Despite evolution in the content of the narratives, the use of selected descriptions of subjective experience as "the document of" underlying psychic entities reveals Freud's persisting influence.

Sample Conversations

The practice of interpreting subjective experience as evidence for underlying realities is beautifully depicted in the article "A Dream While Drowning."[8] In it, Ralph Greenson, a noted psychoanalyst, offered his fellow psychoanalysts clinical data to be taken as evidence confirming the then-popular theories of Margaret Mahler. More to our purposes, the report also illustrates how a naive patient came to reinterpret his experiences by participating in a psychoanalytic conversation. (As background, the reader needs to know that, during World War II, analysts like Greenson served in the armed forces, treating soldiers who had "combat neuroses"—that is, severe psychological reactions to battle experiences. To promote recall of the precipitating trauma, the doctors often used pentothal interviews.) Here is a condensed version of Greenson's report.

> The date was March, 1945. The patient, Frank, had been flown to an air force convalescent hospital from a combat area. His complaint was that, since going on a "bad" mission, his head had been full of repetitious

words or sounds, making him feel as if he "was going nuts." The facts were as follows. Frank had been flying on a mission to take photographs over the South Pacific. He was in the bomb bay of his aircraft, taking photographs, when they were hit by flak. The doors of the bomb bay flew shut, the gasoline tanks were damaged, and gasoline began to pour into and fill up the bomb bay. Frank was unable to climb out, and became overcome by the fumes as the gasoline filled up the bomb bay; he felt paralyzed and that he was drowning.

The repetitious sounds and words began after he had first awakened in a hospital, and had persisted, preventing him from concentrating on anything.

Greenson inquired about the patient's early life, learning among other things that Frank's mother had died when he was quite young, and that he had been raised by his father as an only child on a ranch in Idaho. In order for them to uncover the meaning of the repetitive words, Frank consented to a pentothal interview with Greenson. During part of the interview he said, "I tried to open up the bomb bay, but the gas kept coming in. I lost my mind. Jehosephat. I lost my mind. Amosnell, Domosnell. Amosnell, Domosnell. I kept yelling it . . . but now there was a giant Teddy Bear, but he was a man. And when I got scared, he looked at me and said that I shouldn't worry, he was going to take me into his body, his belly. . . . And he shoved me into his mouth like a candy bar. It took ages and ages and all I heard was Amosnell, Domosnell, Amosnell, Domosnell. And when I woke up I was wrapped in blankets in the hospital and all I kept saying was Amosnell, Domosnell."

Later, Greenson went over various elements of the interview with the patient, asking Frank for his own accounts and personal memories. Frank did not have anything to offer about the Teddy Bear, except that he had slept with one as a child. Greenson said to him, "When kids get real scared, they like to hide someplace where it is safe, like under a blanket. The first safe place a kid experiences is when he is still inside his mother's belly, before he is born. When you were drowning in the gasoline, in the belly of the plane, you must have wished you could get back under those blankets or back inside your mother's belly and feel safe and warm." Frank, Greenson reported, seemed to follow the explanation, and acknowledged it made sense to him. But he still wondered about the Teddy Bear man. Greenson told him that the Teddy Bear man was a combination of his mother and father, the mothering father of his early childhood. "When you got scared to death that you were going to drown, then came the giant Teddy Bear man, who took you back into his belly, where he kept you safe."

According to Greenson, Frank listened to this with open-mouthed wonder and in silence. Then he quietly said that as crazy as it seemed at first, it did make sense. Greenson noted to his readers that the patient put it well by saying, "I dreamed myself back into a safe place."

After this, both of them wondered about the words Amosnell, Domosnell. Greenson suggested they might be foreign words, and asked if Frank's mother had been foreign. Frank thought she had been American, but agreed to write his father and to find out more about her. Greenson saw Frank for supportive psychotherapy, and as they met and talked, the repetitious words began to fade. A letter from Frank's father reported that his wife had been born in Belgium, and although she spoke English, she sang songs in her native language to Frank when he was a baby. She had died when Frank was almost two years old. The father recalled a song that went something like Amosnell, Domosnell. In the meantime, Greenson had reported the phrase to an intelligence officer, and he also received information, to the effect that the words were from a Flemish dialect prevalent in northern Belgium. Their approximate meaning was, "I must hurry, you must hurry." After these confirmations occurred, the words lost their intrusive quality, and Frank sometimes found himself humming them when he was in a good mood.

At the conclusion, Greenson writes, "I submit this fragment of clinical data to indicate how, under conditions of terrifying stress, a person will regress to a symbiotic state of safety, as it has been colored by his personal history. I believe it confirms many of the ideas with which we are now struggling concerning the early relationship of the mothering person and the child."

Whether the story confirms any theory or not, it is fascinating. One of its remarkable elements is the unearthing of the origins of the Flemish phrase. It has been a great problem for an activity that is supposed to depend on historical reconstruction that it virtually never produces confirming data that are not themselves generated by the minds currently at work on the reconstruction. Classical psychoanalysis was premised on the ideal of veridical reconstruction. The chance reconstruction of early language exposure in Greenson's vignette lends authority to the other, more tenuous reconstruction—namely, the discovery of a Mahlerian symbiotic retreat in the dream of the teddy bear.

Note the patient's responses to Greenson's interpretations. He was skeptical, but open-mouthed—one might say, ready to take it in. Certainly, it was unlikely that he had ever heard talk like this before. But of course, he had never had an experience like this traumatic one or his subsequent illness. He was frightened, confused, and in need of help. The doctor was an authority, a kind person who had spent time getting to know him, and someone who in addition had carried out a dramatic procedure, with a substance (Greenson tells us) known to servicemen as "flak juice." When this doctor told Frank the meaning of his dream of the teddy bear, Frank did the natural, human thing—

he took up the conversation. His rephrasing of the interpretation in his own words was greeted with satisfaction by Greenson, as evidence of Frank's acceptance of it, and therefore of its correctness. Now they were talking.

We do not have an explanation for the fact that the repeated phrase eventually extinguished itself. The classical explanation is that a symptom fades once its unconscious roots are revealed. But Greenson seems to be hinting at something different. He notes that he established a relationship of a supportive kind with the young serviceman. After the dramatic discovery of the origin of "Amosnell, Domosnell," the phrase might have become emblematic of this relationship, which helped Frank to make sense of a bewildering experience. It tagged an experience in which something alien had been made over into a recognizable part of himself. It became associated, in fact, with his better moods.

On several levels, then, this story is about producing something as evidence for a theory. Greenson convinced Frank that his experience was evidence for a longing to return to the safety of his mother's womb. Frank, for his part, participated in constructing his experience in this way, and so it was co-constructed by them both. Greenson put the story forward to his fellow analysts as evidence for the truth of the Mahlerian theory of symbiosis. Such a vignette is part of the larger set of experiences by which analysts are brought into the belief system of psychoanalytic theory.

We now turn to a second, more modern psychoanalytic conversation, a fragment of a psychoanalytic session. The patient, a man who had been in analysis for several years, recounted a dream, and some thoughts about the dream, to the analyst (the dream is in italics). In the fragment there is a reference to a song, "Duke of Earl," which had figured prominently in the analytic work some months previously.

Patient: *I am at a feast, in a mansion. For entertainment, there is a whole basketball team there, playing. They are a championship team, from Duke.* (He pauses.)

I don't want to know the actual truth about this, but I am wondering if you have any connection with Duke, since you are from the South.

I am at a table, ready to eat the feast, but Sarah's father is also there, looking stern and authoritarian.

Duke . . . reminds me of "Duke of Earl." (pause) Oh, I just remembered that Sarah's father's middle name is Earl! That is pretty amazing, that the dream linked "Duke" and "Earl" this way. Did my unconscious do that? If it did, how can we use that to help me feel better?

Analyst: Actually, I don't believe in the unconscious.

Patient: *Now* you tell me!

(Both laugh.)

Analyst: I wonder whether something happened here in this room, to make that link.

Patient: It's very interesting that you don't believe in the unconscious—I never liked the unconscious anyway . . . (pause). Do you know what actually happened while I was telling you the dream? As soon as I mentioned "Duke" to you, I imagined that you were off in your own narcissistic world, thinking about yourself. That's when I thought of "Earl," someone arrogant. Probably if Sarah's father hadn't been in the dream, it would have gone in some other direction. Anyway, I'm not sure her father had that name, it might have been her brother. Yes, I made the link myself.

(The patient went on to contrast the idea of being a passive mouthpiece for his "unconscious" with the idea that he was creating meanings actively, finding much hope in this latter view of himself. The analyst expressed a positive interest in this turn of events in their conversation.)

At its most superficial level, this is a conversation in which the pair (my patient and myself) switches from an isolated-mind perspective (my patient's unconscious "did it") to an interactional perspective. At this level, the contrast between the isolated mind and the relational experience can be seen in my patient's amended description of what had happened. Even when I was saying nothing, as he was telling and commenting on the dream he took my silence to *mean something*—namely, narcissistic self-preoccupation. Thus, his subsequent thoughts were responsive to the experience of being in the company of a narcissist. Interaction was being represented at every moment, whether there was talk or not.

Stepping outside my patient's account of his associations and moving to the level of the conversation itself, his dialogic reactions and adaptations to my unanticipated disclosure and suggestion *also* illustrate the dynamic nature of the relational situation. The psychoanalyst Christopher Bollas has called the analytic process "a successional interplay of idiom elements" and has dubbed "subject relations theory" the attention to "the interplay of two human sensibilities, who together create environments unique to their cohabitation."[9] It could be said that I exposed my relational theory, which was part of *my* idiom at that moment. In the new light of this exposure, my patient reconstructed his own experience of the previous association, and thereby developed a new facet of his experience of self. This "evidence" for a more active self was then also accepted by me, placing the finishing touch on a co-constructed story of subjective experience. In the conversation we see, too, some mutual play with the frame, both in my revelation and in his "*Now* you tell me!"—which can be seen as both a quip and a remonstrance. These are aspects of the extended, performative conversation.

What about the dream? Dreams historically have a privileged role in the psychoanalytic conversation, in that they are treated as communicative acts on the same level as other communicative acts. We know that the physiological substrate of dreaming is random activation of neural assemblies distributed throughout the brain. It is difficult to produce a seamless narrative from odds and ends—but preliminary sense-making appears to take place in the course of dreaming itself, through the overlay of primitive temporal frames (such as "and then...") and causal explanations ("because").[10] Dreams undergo further narrative revision when they are recalled on awakening and still further revision when they are recounted. These successive narrative constructions are aided by the fact that the very neural assemblies that encode parts of the previous day's experiences are activated in the dream to yield fragmented and disordered impressions of those experiences. Thus, some parts of the dream at least seem to point in an obscure way to the experiences of the dreamer the day before. The fragmentary images in dreams become narrative "emblems": "There is one overriding property that all such emblems share that makes them different from logical propositions. Impenetrable to both inference and induction, they resist logical procedures for establishing what they *mean*. They must, as we say, be *interpreted*."[11]

Dreams are like the blowholes found near ancient Indian dwellings in northern Arizona. Blowholes are small natural openings in the ground, connecting underground caverns to the outside. At various times, because of pressure differentials above and below ground, air moves through the hole, making resonant sounds. To the humans nearby, these are not random sounds—they are the mutterings of spirits, intended communications. The holes "talk." In the same way, dreams "talk." In particular cultural contexts, such as soothsaying or psychoanalysis, random brain noise is collaboratively construed as meaningful in particular ways. Dreams present themselves as strings of meaning elaborated in a social setting in order to communicate and *to be responded to with further narratives.* In psychoanalysis, these further narratives are called interpretations. A dream and its interpretation constitute a conversational exchange. Such a responsive sequence illustrates the general tendency of narratives to attract, and become linked with, other narratives.

That No-Man's-Land of Undiluted Humanity

We have seen how a patient's expressive peculiarities, momentary or chronic, are assumed by psychoanalysts to be documents of underlying psychic configurations. In the logically circular process of analytic "exploration," such underlying configurations are both presumed and discovered in the patient's communications.

The process takes place in two steps. First, significant expressive moments are registered. At the heart of the psychoanalytic enterprise, I believe, are momentary suspensions of the documentary method, times when the analyst suspends belief in the patient's "self" and registers his or her signs simply as signs in relation to other signs. During these moments of suspension, the irregularities, discontinuities, or other specific arrangements of the whole pattern constituted by the patient's emerging performance and narrative become transiently manifest. In a succeeding step, in most analyses, the documentary method reasserts inself: The analyst draws in the just-perceived forms as evidence for something else, something present but unseen. As evidence that my characterization of this sequence is accurate, I submit the following account by the psychoanalyst Evelyne Schwaber, in which the analyst first selected fragments from the unfolding performance, and then took them as indicators of something else.

"Ms. E . . . arrived at an hour which I had rescheduled and told me that she had mistakenly arranged for a dental appointment at the same time. She was *'certain'* the error must have meaning. Noticing the emphasis, I asked, 'What makes you certain?'"

The patient answered the question and continued, but began to speak more vaguely and haltingly. Noticing this, the analyst inquired about it. The patient then said that the analyst's question had made her feel as others' responses to her in her childhood had also made her feel—namely, stupid. In response to this feeling, the patient had lost her sense of certainty and confidence, just as she had done formerly. Summarizing this sequence of events, Schwaber wrote: "We . . . seek to elucidate meanings in minute, often scarcely registered cues, affective—including tonal—expressions, and invite the patient to observe and bring them into awareness. For such communications may serve as cogent carriers of what is yet unconscious."[12] That is, a communicative nuance was detected, and then explained by reference to an underlying unconscious determinant.

Let us return to the critical moments around the time the analyst asked her question, examining them still more closely. Schwaber wrote that she had felt herself becoming inattentive and disengaged from the patient: It was this that drew her to notice and inquire about the vague quality of the patient's speech. During the moments of sensing her own and her patient's flatness, it seems the analyst abandoned the documentary method. She suspended the kind of thought that construes surface events as documents of underlying realities. In doing this, she was able to stay on the surface of the communicative stream of signs, and feel, then respond to, its *form*. It is as though a patient's communications are a kind of tapestry: The analyst who is attentive to the weaving notices places where the pattern changes.

At this point, the second step was taken—that is, the documentary method was resumed. After noticing the quality of the patient's speech, Schwaber remarked on it; in response, the patient told her more. At precisely this point, joint construction of the patient's history began. But why is the documentary method customarily resorted to at such moments? It may be because psychoanalysts confuse the documentary method, which is everyday practice, with the scientific method. They believe that the observation of a local idiomatic event is like the observation of precipitate in a glass beaker—that it indicates the presence of some other, invisible elements acting according to natural laws. The analyst's remark and the patient's further response lead to their co-construction of these supposed underlying realities.

In fact, however, co-construction of supposed underlying realities is elective in a psychoanalytic treatment. Psychoanalysts and their patients could dispense with the historical reconstruction that normally occurs at this juncture, contenting themselves with the extension of communication that is taking place between them. That is, if they are willing to be radical about it, psychoanalysts could just as well abandon the documentary method altogether. Instead, they could understand psychoanalysis as a conversation that, more urgently than any other, forces the participants to strive to achieve a common system of signs. In the process of this striving, each will inevitably experience moments when the idiom of the other is somehow strange.

In a psychoanalysis so conceived, the analyst's reflection on the patient's stream of signs, and for that matter the patient's reflections on the analyst's, yield again and again the same discovery. What they discover is simply that individual sign systems are *composed*, each with its own particular aesthetic. The selves of both patient and analyst *are* these sign patterns, and nothing more—although believing literally in the person concept may make us think there is something more. Robert Perinbanayagam writes:

> The self has only an epistemological status and has no ontology that is independent of the methods used to describe it or show it or think it: it is coterminous with the terminology and iconography used in each situation and context in which it is presented, described or conceived. Such

methods, however, and the terminologies that issue from them are *reflexively potent*: they become signs that project inwards to the mind of the initiating subject and outwards into the thinking process of others. The fundamental status of self, then, is that of a sign that produces a double interpretant—one by a thinking process and the other by the thinking process of another person.[13]

The suspension of the documentary method has in fact been hinted at by several psychoanalysts, often in ways that sound cryptic because they are outside mainstream thought. Wilfred Bion wrote, for example:

> Every session attended by the psychoanalyst must have no history and no future. . . . What is "known" about the patient is of no further consequence: it is either false or irrelevant. If it is "known" by patient and analyst, it is obsolete.
> . . . The psychoanalyst should aim at achieving a state of mind so that at every session he feels he has not seen the patient before.[14]

Hellmuth Kaiser movingly described a personal journey from classical assumptions to a reconceptualization of the therapeutic core of psychoanalytic work.[15] Summarizing his reflections, he wrote:

> In other words, the theoretically prescribed goal of the psychoanalytic procedure (thought of more or less as "making the unconscious conscious") required, as technical means, that therapist and patient meet regularly over a long period of time under conditions which favored, to a certain extent, real communication between them.
> . . . The postulated condition that the therapist, by dint of his personality, maintains a communicative attitude towards the patient is much more radical than the words seem to convey. . . . [The therapist] has no handrail, no mapped track or charted course to follow. The more of a therapist he is, the more he moves out from any of the hundreds and thousands of patterns which shape the different types of interaction between people and which form our social life in the word's broadest meaning.
> . . . One feels a bit freer to leave the rules behind and venture in—well, what could I call it?—that no-man's-land of undiluted humanity!

Psychoanalytic narratives have been mistaken in the past for technical knowledge of real entities such as "drives," "objects," "self-objects," "motivational systems," and "schemas." But change in psychoanalytic theory is not like progress in scientific understanding. Instead, it is like the movement from Impressionism to Cubism. No metapsychology is more true than any other—there are only greater and lesser masters, and more and less interesting narrative innovations. Psychoanalytic theories (drive psychology, ego psychology, object relations theory, self psychology) continually put new narratives at the disposal of practitioners, adding to the potential richness of the dialogue for both patients and other practitioners. When during a session the analyst uses such theories to infer the presence of real entities that determine the patient's communications, however, the analyst risks losing his or her immersion in the stream of signs, immersion in both his or her own and the patient's "undiluted humanity."

In other chapters we developed the idea that "person" is a consensual affair established through the exchange of signs. A patient in a real sense exists *more* as a person in an analytic conversation than in any other conversation, because here the stream of acts and stories is registered and responded to more thoroughly than anywhere else. The willing response to this stream of signals is the analyst's part; the willing generation of the stream is the patient's part. Generating and responding to acts and stories is what human beings are all about. To live fully in the communicative world is indeed to experience undiluted humanity. The psychoanalytic pair, in their best moments, have that privilege.

10

Exile's End

The natural sciences, the sciences of physics and chemistry that describe living matter, are concerned with causes. I have used a natural-science framework to describe the evolved structures and functions of individual brains. Because of the social capabilities that human brains possess, two or more brains together can produce and receive signals, giving rise to public signs—or meaning. The zone of publicly communicated signs occupies a transitional area between what we can describe using the language of natural science and what we may call the language of mind. The language of mind, as we saw, is primarily concerned with the actions of persons and deals with reasons rather than with causes.

The languages of mind and natural science are related in several ways. First, the latter can explain the origins of the former. We use the language of science when we describe how our brains evolved to engage in conversation, to generate representations of "person" with attendant representations of subjective mental life, and to create a superordinate moral-social order that organizes the perceived activities of persons. Second, as a result of these capacities, our brains traffic in entities that can only be described using the language of mind. The performances and narratives taking place in the public, communicative arena produce a myriad of culturally specific social objects—shoulds and oughts, reasons and motivations. People in social groups are both natural receptacles and spawning grounds for these objects, which fill conversation, person, and the moral-social order with specific, situated forms. Because the social mind doubles back in this way onto the individual, my talk obeys the rules for middle-class American conversation rather than the rules for Maasai conversation, and I understand the shoulds and oughts in narratives regarding academic hierarchy as opposed to those in narratives regarding warriorhood, for example. The person concept illustrates this trafficking especially well: The concept of subjectivity springs from the brain's mindmaking specialization described in the first four chapters, but it is given flesh by performances and narratives—as described in chapters 6 and 7—that yield culturally specific forms of "self" or "person." The brain's capabilities are vessels for living cultural forms.

On the other hand, there is a way in which the languages of mind and natural science appear to coincide, but in fact do not. The language of mind often invokes "mental" entities—for example, "willpower," "emotion," "superego," "boredom," "reasoning." Such entities become social objects by being subscribed to publicly in performances and narratives, which, as we saw, create strong consensual convictions of reality. These convictions may make us feel that we are talking of empirically established entities. Of the words just listed, some are obviously just our "manner of speaking," whereas others may be erroneously accepted as scientifically established. The word "emotion," as we saw, has been erroneously accepted as a valid category in neuroscience. It is one example of a spurious interaction between everyday mentalistic language and the language of science, an interaction that can mislead both laypeople and scientists.

Why is this interaction so difficult to detect? Disentangling the language of natural science from the everyday language we are accustomed to, which refers to reasons and mental states, is not just a matter of being hardnosed and analytical. Thinking that is concerned purely with empirically testable statements about causes is something scientists aspire to, and something they achieve occasionally, but it is not a natural mode for human beings. One can decide to be hardnosed—but how does one know if one's ideas are actually contaminated by beliefs imported from the world of everyday understanding? Everyday beliefs do not announce themselves as nonscientific. Far from it: Their hallmark is that they seem so obvious as to be beyond questioning.

The sociologist Emanuel Schegloff has used the term "vernacular culture" to describe the system of everyday beliefs to which we all subscribe whether we know it or not. He has likened the vernacular culture to the world of microbes. To think scientifically requires a sterile conceptual field and continuous vigilance to keep the ubiquitous vernacular "organisms" at bay. This is a useful image for several reasons. It reminds us that we achieve scientific thought only with effort, just as it takes energy and resources to remove bacteria from areas where surgery is to be performed. Furthermore, both sterile fields and scientific thought do not remain uninfiltrated for very long—they are always under pressure from encroaching contamination.

The image also suggests what we might gain by studying the mechanisms of everyday thought. Just as understanding deoxyribonucleic acid (DNA) has given us a great deal of control over the world of bacteria and other organisms, understanding conversation should allow us to appreciate how the vernacular culture replicates itself everywhere there are human beings, ingeniously colonizing human imagination—including scientific imagination. In the same way that a virus can excerpt and incorporate snippets of another organism's DNA, vernacular culture can take up bits of science and incorporate them into its own system. Moreover, it can stealthily permeate whole disciplines, causing people to carry out practices that are extensions of vernacular culture masquerading as science. Only by looking to the criteria of prediction and control on the one hand, and by detecting everyday practices like the use of the documentary method on the other, can we tease scientific and everyday thought apart. Whether we seek to separate them or merely to contemplate their intermingling, however, we can appreciate both scientific and everyday thought as remarkable, if quite different, human achievements.[1]

Let us now retrace our journey. We saw that the concept of the isolated mind has a history. Beginning in the Enlightenment period, the idea took hold that nature can be known through the methods of empirical science, methods that in principle are free from social influence. The human mind became a knowing mind, splendidly isolated from other minds, a "mirror of nature." Thus did our Robinson Crusoe set sail.

In modern times, neuroscientists continued to use this metaphor of the mind to structure brain research, for, because of the very nature of vernacular ideas—especially ideas made venerable by centuries of use—the concept was never scrutinized. If one treated Robinson Crusoe as entirely asocial, however, severe problems would arise in explaining his diaries, his prayers, and all his ideas. This is exactly what ultimately happened in cognitive neuroscience: Because asocial brains are actually mindless, it was logically impossible to make the leap from the isolated brain to the mind.

In the seventeenth century, if there had been cognitive neuroscientists, they might have tried to finesse the problem by declaring that the brain simply must produce the vernacular categories they knew—such as religious thought and diary-writing—"must" because otherwise they would have been forced into mind–brain dualism. Being members of their societies and thinking along the only lines available to them, they would have designed and interpreted their brain experiments according to extant vernacular categories of the mind. If they had had brain scanners, they might have done experiments on the neural basis of godly behavior and prayer. And if these hypothetical scientists were very industrious, producing vast quantities of data packaged into avalanches of scholarly articles, the laypersons of their time would surely have been forgiven for concluding that the major mysteries of the brain had been solved—as attested to by the fact that the brain apparently produced just the things they expected, such as godly behavior, diary-writing, and so on. As long as they remained oblivious to the fact that their own community had created these categories, it would not occur to them to ask how their brains had worked together to create just this community of thought, and the muddle would go on and on. The vernacular nature of mental categories, together with the social nature of the brain, would remain equally and simultaneously invisible.

I have tried in this book to render them both visible. My aim has been to end Crusoe's strange exile and send him back to his community—where he belongs.

In attempting to adhere to the language of natural science I may have seemed to discard mentalist language in favor of the kind of behaviorism that psychology abandoned rather triumphantly a generation ago—for example, by using phrases like "disposition to act" instead of "feeling." My emphasis has been on public behavior as opposed to isolated behavior, however—and this is a key difference. Symbolic interactionism, unlike antimentalist, isolated behaviorism, offers an account of mind, which is that mind is a public system of signs and behavior. As we saw, this theory is not new, but it has tended to be studied by sociologists rather than by neuroscientists. We can say that George Herbert Mead, who developed the theory, set the sails on the ship that is taking Crusoe home.

Other ideas in this book are also decades old. The idea that it is an error to try to collapse entities that belong to the language of mind into the natural sciences—the brain—has been expressed before. Wittgenstein, for example, held it to be a form of occultism to take psychological terms as documents of underlying neural entities. Elaborating on this idea, the philosopher Norman Malcolm wrote:

> In our discourse with one another we make innumerable references to things and situations. We employ concepts, descriptions, representations. We express impressions, feelings, expectations, doubts, anxieties. The idea that all of these ingredients of thinking are packed into that narrow space inside the skull, fills one with amazement. It provides the thrill of the incomprehensible—just as magic does![2]

Eschewing magic, and finding out what really does go on in "that narrow space inside the skull," is the goal of neuroscience.

Many scientists suspect that what goes on in the brain has very little relation to the everyday language of the mental. At the same time, they intuitively appreciate that our everyday understandings make us what we are, that we live for the most part in the language of the mind. What I have tried to do in this book is to convey the richness and power of everyday interaction, showing how it produces the language of the mind, reasons, and selves. In contrast to contemporary cognitive neuroscience, which views the mind as a kind of closet with entities like emotion, linguistic rules, and memory arranged inside, I take mind to be irreducibly transactional. Rather than something packed inside a solitary skull, it is a dynamic entity defined by its transactions with the rest of the world: Like industrial regions, theater districts, and shipping ports, minds are best characterized by reference to the larger forms of life in which they play a part. Just as gold's value derives not from its chemical composition but from public agreement, the essence of thought is not its isolated neural basis, but its social use.

Notes

CHAPTER 1

1. Excerpted from Feinberg and Shapiro (1989, pp. 40–41).

2. Excerpt from Kanner (1944, p. 216).

3. See Strawson (1959) and Ayer (1963).

4. Term taken from Harré (1993). The relation between person and social order is expressed by Douglas (1992, p.60) as follows: "The community is the locus of ideology connecting the idea of the person to the culture which its members are making."

5. Jackendoff (1987, p. 261) calls the aspects of images or words that we experience "intermediate level representations," and notes, "One cannot choose not to organize visual input along the lines specified by the visual system, except by closing one's eyes. Likewise, one cannot hear a speech stream as mere sound, especially in a language one understands."

We can think of the semantic aspect as referring to the level of categorization that is significant for *action*, where the array of possible actions belongs to a social system. In other words—as the philosopher Wittgenstein argued—the meaning of a word derives from the system of public uses to which it is put. The equation of semantics with behavioral disposition was made, for example, by Quine (1969).

6. Bruner (1990, p. 39). Although it has its uses, the term "folk psychology" is a bit troublesome. Phrases that also use the word "folk," such as folk dancing and folk art, connote quaint simplicity: Folk productions seem almost to announce themselves by their naive style. Our everyday beliefs, including our everyday notions of mind, in contrast, do not announce themselves as nonscientific, are quite sophisticated, and are much more pervasive than we realize. These features of everyday thought, and its relation to scientific thought, are discussed in more detail in the final chapter of the book.

7. Silva and Leong (1991, pp. 103–104).

8. A comprehensive classification scheme, followed in the present discussion, has been put forward in Silva, Leong and Shaner (1990). See also Signer (1987) and Silva, Leong, and Shaner (1991).

9. These examples were taken from Ardila, Botero, Gomez, and Quijano (1988). Other cases in this section, and reviews of the role of brain injury in misidentification syndromes, are found in Silva, et al. (1991); Ardila and Rosseli (1988); Joseph (1985); Malliaras, Kossovitsa, and Christodoulou (1978); and Silva, Leong, and Weinstock (1991). A neurocognitive account for some misidentification syndromes has been offered in Young (1992). For experiments and discussion regarding right hemisphere involvement in Capgras syndrome, see Ellis et al. (1993).

10. The neurologist Antonio Damasio (1994, pp. 242–243) gave a related but somewhat different account of the way body and mind are connected. His account addresses the sense of subjectivity—that is, the attribution of mind to oneself—but not the attribution of mind to other bodies. It derives subjectivity from representations of one's own body as it responds to sensory influences. Damasio's account is consistent with the clinical findings discussed in this chapter—namely, that brain lesions affecting pathways arising in the parietal lobes (where bodily sensations are registered) and converging in the temporal lobes impair the sense of self. Assuming that Damasio's and my own account are roughly accurate, it becomes a problem to explain why many patients with disruptions of subjectivity also experience disruptions of the perception of *others'* bodies and minds. A solution may be in sight. Giacomo Rizzolatti and his co-workers have recently discovered neurons in monkeys that respond both to the animals' own hand movements and to the identical hand movements the animal observes being performed by others (Gallese, Fadiga, Fogassi, Rizzolatti, 1996). Their findings raise the possibility that the perception of our own bodies and the creation of our own subjectivities is accomplished by the same brain circuits that represent other bodies and minds.

11. From Ramachandran, V. (1990). Interactions between motion, depth, color and form: The utilitarian theory of perception. In C. Blakemore (ed.), *Vision: Coding and Efficiency*. Cambridge: Cambridge University Press, pp. 346–360. Copyright © 1990 Cambridge University Press. Reprinted by permission of Cambridge University Press.

12. For definitions and descriptions of autism reviewed in this section, see Wing (1988a, 1988b). For discussions of autism's neural bases, see Brothers (1990); Baron-Cohen and Ring (1994); Baron-Cohen (1995); Piven, et al. (1990); and Courchesne (1987).

13. The developmental linguist John Locke pointed out that, for the young child, intonated adult voices are carriers not only of expressiveness, but also of precursor linguistic information in the form of vowel sounds, which will eventually be important for discriminating words. Movements of the face and voice, he wrote, "attract and sustain the infant's attention to what will become

a linguistically important stream of cues" (Locke, 1993, p. 46). There are two developmental links between perceiving faces and voices at first, and language subsequently. First, facial and vocal expressiveness is interesting to infants, acting as a "hook" to prepare the developing visual and auditory systems of the infants for language receptiveness. Second, the child's perception of linguistic utterances is overlaid onto mechanisms already in place for *perceiving and responding to expressive beings* (see Locke, 1993, p. 83, on "the infralinguistic core" of vocal messages). Understanding beings who signal their intentions and dispositions nonlinguistically is essential scaffolding for the subsequent understanding of linguistic acts.

14. For infant attention to social features discussed in this section, see Goren, Sarty, and Wu (1975); Meltzoff and Moore (1977); Field, Woodson, Greenberg and Cohen (1982); Aronson and Rosenbloom (1971); Haith, Bergman and Moore (1977); and Fernald, et al. (1989). For our sensivitity to facial expressions, see Etcoff and Magee (1992). This research is discussed further in chapter 8. Regarding lipreading, see Campbell (1992).

15. The experimental findings summarized here appear in Corina, Vaid, and Bellugi (1992); Wittling and Roschmann (1993); Cicone, Wapner, and Gardner (1980); Campbell, et al. (1990); Campbell, Landis and Regard (1986); Ross (1981); Ross and Mesulam (1979). Activity of the right hemisphere during naming was demonstrated by Salmelin, Hari, Lounasmaa, and Sams (1994).

16. Weeks and Hobson (1987).

17. Autistic children's inattentiveness to the upper half of the face was shown by Langdell (1978). Their achievements and limitations in understanding gaze direction are documented in Baron-Cohen (1989, 1995) and Baron-Cohen and Cross (1992). Their inability to structure conversations is reported in Baron-Cohen (1988) and Tager-Flusberg, et al. (1990).

18. The findings in this paragraph and the next were reported by Attwood, Frith, and Hermelin (1988); Yirmiya, Sigman, Kasari, and Mundy (1992); and Tager-Flusberg (1992).

19. Fay (1979).

20. See Goffman (1967, 1974, p. 527). Harré (1984, pp. 64–65) wrote: "Just as ordinary things and events have locations in the grids of Newtonian space and time, so commitments, avowals, rememberings and feelings have locations at persons in the psychosocial array. I take the array of persons as a primary human reality. I take the conversations in which those persons are engaged as completing the primary structure, bringing into being social and psychological reality. . . . People and their modes of talk are made by and for social orders, and social orders are people in conversation."

21. Regarding savant capabilities, see Treffert (1989). Frith's quotation is taken from her excellent book on autism (Frith, 1989, p. 108).

22. When there is loss of a sensory capacity resulting from peripheral damage, the brain reallocates sensory areas to other modalities (Neville, 1990). For a review of autistic-like features in blindness, see Hobson (1990).

CHAPTER 2

1. The studies of children's understanding of mental and nonmental representations mentioned here are from Wimmer and Perner (1983); Zaitchik (1990); and Sullivan and Winner (1993). See also Fodor (1992) and Wimmer and Weichbold (1994).

2. Excerpted from Whiten and Byrne (1989, p. 31).

3. The term "theory of mind" was coined by Premack and Woodruff (1978). Studies and discussions of "theory of mind" in nonhuman primates referred to here are from Premack (1988); Cheney and Seyfarth (1990); and Kummer, Dasser, and Hoyningen-Huene (1990). The chimpanzee experiments were conducted by Premack, whose conclusions are generally supported by the more recent work of Povinelli and Eddy (1996). See Cheney, Seyfarth and Smuts (1986), regarding the disparity between social and nonsocial intelligence in monkeys.

4. For these evolutionary arguments, see Humphrey (1984); Brothers (1990); and Allman and McGuinness (1988).

5. Karmiloff-Smith, Klima, Bellugi, Grant, and Baron-Cohen (1995).

6. The findings referred to in this section are from Baron-Cohen (1992); Leekam and Perner (1991); Charman and Baron-Cohen (1995); and Tager-Flusberg (1993). It should be noted that not all mental states cause difficulty: Autistic persons understand seeing, some simple emotions, and desires. They generally do not use terms referring to mental states in their spontaneous talk, however.

7. The excerpt is from Kanner (1943, p. 250). See also Hobson (1990). The experimental findings are published in Hobson (1986); Weeks and Hobson (1987); Sigman, Kasari, Kwon and Yirmiya (1992); and Yirmiya, Sigman, Kasari, and Mundy (1992).

8. Brothers (1990); and Brothers and Ring (1992). See also Brothers (1995).

9. Structured interactions are generally made possible by rule systems. For example, the shared rule systems of language—grammar—make informative oral communication possible. In this passage I am suggesting that a small set of rules, a kind of grammar, emerged as a result of changes in our brains. This grammar is composed of loci of subjectivity (first, second, and third person) and unique identities (one per body). Just as language organizes the stream of vocal sounds we make and hear, person-rules organize the stream of social gestures we produce and interpret.

We follow those rules, but we can imagine other rules. In "thought experiments," philosophers have imagined variations of this grammar—such as walking, talking human bodies devoid of subjective experience—in order to try to explain consciousness. Such experiments have not generated much real progress. It is like imagining one player of a Monopoly game moving his piece counterclockwise instead of clockwise: this cannot help us understand why players generally move their pieces clockwise.

10. Brothers (1994).

11. Patterson and Baddeley (1977).

12. Excerpts from pp. 31 and 67 of Bruce, V. (1988). *Recognizing Faces*. East Sussex, UK: Lawrence Erlbaum. Copyright © Lawrence Erlbaum Associates, Ltd. Reprinted by permission of Lawrence Erlbaum Associates, Ltd., Hove, U.K.

CHAPTER 3

1. *Primate* refers to the order of mammals containing monkeys, apes, and humans. Hereafter, we shall use "nonhuman primate" to refer to monkeys and apes.

Neurons are the individual cells of which the brain is composed. Neurons are electrically excitable, and can communicate changes in electrical potentials with other neurons, via the actions of chemicals called neurotransmitters. Neurons communicate with other neurons throughout the brain by "firing," that is, by producing action potentials. These signals travel, like phone messages down a wire, along fine extensions called axons that may reach many millimeters into the brain to make contact with other neurons. It is through the organized activity of billions of neurons that the brain does its work. In this book, the terms "cell" and "neuron" are used interchangeably.

Cortex (cortical; *adj*; cortices, *pl.*) is a sheet of neurons about 2 millimeters thick that forms the surface of the brain. The cortex of the human brain is highly folded, giving rise to furrows (sulcus, sulci, *pl.*) where the cortex folds in and disappears from view, and the rounded ridges (gyrus, gyri, *pl.*) of cortex that we see when we look at a whole brain.

2. Reports of these important early findings can be found in Barlow (1953); Barlow, Fitzhigh, and Kuffler (1957); Hubel (1959); and Hubel and Wiesel (1959).

3. Excerpted from Defoe (1719/1957, p. 203).

4. The excerpt comes from Gross, Rocha-Miranda, and Bender (1972, pp. 103–104). Gross's co-workers during these experiments also included Tom Albright, Charles Bruce, and Robert Desimone. A brief published report of the hand-selective cell first appeared in 1969 (Gross, Bender, Rocha-Miranda, 1969).

5. This is explained in Eichenbaum (1993).

6. The excerpt is from Bruce, Desimone, and Gross (1981, p. 374).

7. Sanghera, Rolls, and Roper-Hall (1979).

8. The studies referred to in this section are reported in Desimone, Albright, Gross, and Bruce (1984); Rolls (1981); Brothers and Ring (1993); Brothers, Ring, and Kling (1990); Leonard, Rolls, Wilson, and Baylis (1985); and Nakamura, Mikami, and Kubota (1992).

9. The notion of linking regions in the brain was spelled out in Damasio (1989b).

10. The studies referred to in this section are reported in Baylis, Rolls, and Leonard (1985); Bruce, Desimone, and Gross (1981); Desimone, Albright,

Gross, and Bruce (1984); Leonard, Rolls, Wilson, and Baylis (1985); and Perrett, Rolls, and Caan (1979, 1982).

11. Rolls (1995).

12. Studies of neurons that respond to distinguishing physical features of faces include Yamane, Kaji, and Kawano (1988); Baylis, Rolls, and Leonard (1985); Leonard, Rolls, Wilson, and Baylis (1985); Young and Yamane (1992); Nahm (1994); and Nahm, Albright, and Amaral (1991).

13. Studies of neurons that respond to facial expressions referred to in this section are reported in Hasselmo, Rolls, and Baylis (1989); Perrett, et al. (1984); Perrett and Mistlin (1990); and Nakamura, Mikami, and Kubota (1992).

14. Perrett has contributed greatly to our understanding of how the brain responds to gaze direction in others. He suggests that gaze- and head-orientation-selective neurons might encode the direction of the stimulus animal's attention, and notes that this is a simple kind of mental state. See Perrett et al. (1985); and Perrett, Heitanen, Oram, and Benson (1992) for key research findings in this area.

15. Oram and Perrett (1994); Perrett, Harries, Benson, Chitty, and Mistlin (1990); and Perrett, Harries, Chitty, and Mistlin (1990).

16. Brothers, Ring, and Kling (1990); Brothers and Ring (1993).

17. Baizer, Ungerleider and Desimone (1991); Boussaoud, Ungerleider and Desimone (1990).

18. Brothers and Ring (1993). The first individual was the female head of the laboratory and known to the animal. The second was an unknown male from another department. The other two individuals, to whom the cell did not respond, were the male laboratory technician (familiar to the animal), and an unfamiliar female. Thus the identity response was not due either to familiarity or to gender.

19. Analyses of the role of the anterior temporal lobes in producing the behavioral changes described here can be traced in Brown and Schäfer (1888); Klüver and Bucy (1937, 1939); Schreiner and Kling (1956); Weiskrantz (1956); and Downer (1962).

20. Original reports on the effects of amygdala lesions in a variety of species can be found in Schreiner and Kling (1953); Dicks, Myers, and Kling (1969); Kling, Lancaster, and Benitone (1970); and Kling, Dicks, and Gurowitz (1969). They are also surveyed in Kling and Brothers (1992).

21. The importance of recognizing species diversity, as opposed to using the brain of one nonhuman primate species as a model for all primate brains, including human ones, has been pointed out in Preuss (1994).

22. Changes in brain chemistry caused by social isolation in monkeys are reported in Kling et al. (1992).

23. Regarding the role of the orbital frontal cortex in monkey social behavior see Raleigh (1976) and Raleigh and Steklis (1981). The proposed brain system for social bonding is described in Kling and Steklis (1976).

24. Further details on the effects of brain stimulation can be found in Penfield and Rasmussen (1950); Penfield and Roberts (1959); and Ojemann (1990).

25. The stimulation experiments referred to are found in Kaada (1951); Jürgens and Ploog (1970); Raleigh and Steklis (1981); Robinson (1967); Robinson and Mishkin (1968); and Ursin (1972).

CHAPTER 4

1. The excerpts are from Gloor (1986, p. 164).

2. A review of the effects of temporal lobe stimulation by two of its pioneers can be found in Penfield and Rasmussen (1950). Explanations for the quality of the recalled scenes can be found in Gloor (1986, 1990).

3. The excerpt is from Gloor (1986, p. 165).

4. Feedback from the amygdala and other regions may occur either directly, through their neural projections back to sensory areas, or indirectly in the somatic states that amygdala activity has set into motion. Such states are a source of sensory input to the brain. Representations of somatic states may be juxtaposed to representations from the external world, as described by Damasio (1994), in such a way as to bias their significance.

5. Dennett (1991, pp. 385–386).

6. Kirkpatrick (1985).

7. Gerber (1985).

8. From Tranel, D., Hyman, B. (1990). Neuropsychological correlates of bilateral amygdala damage. *Archives of Neurology, 47*; 349–355. Copyright © 1990, American Medical Association.

9. The deficits seen in the two patients with localized amygdala damage are described in Tranel and Hyman (1990); Adolphs, Tranel, Damasio, and Damasio (1994, 1995); Young et al. (1995). Other patients who did not show the same deficits are described in Hamann et al. (1996). Complementing these discoveries in patients with amygdala damage, researchers have recently shown that amygdala activity in normal subjects is affected by the sight of facial expressions: Neural acitivity—especially in the left amygdala—increases when an individual sees pictures of fearful faces, but not when he or she sees faces with happy expressions. See Morris, Frith, Perrett, Rowland, Young, Calder and Dolan (1996).

10. The details of EVR's difficulties may be found in Eslinger and Damasio (1985); Damasio, Tranel, and Damasio (1990b); Saver and Damasio (1991); and Damasio (1994). The case of the woman with anterior cingulate damage is reported in Damasio and van Hoesen (1983).

11. The findings are reported in Fried, Mateer, Ojemann, Wohns, and Fedio (1982).

12. Primary sensory cortex is cortex that receives direct inputs from sensory organs. Neurons in primary sensory cortex send connections to association cortex, which is presumed to carry out higher levels of processing. Neurons in association cortices may receive inputs from primary cortices serving more than one kind of sensory modality (for example, vision and touch). For changes in the amygdala during evolution, see Stephan, Frahm, and Baron (1987). Regarding changes in cortex, see Passingham (1975).

13. The extensive connections of amygdala with cortex are discussed in Price and Amaral (1981) and in Amaral, Price, Pitkanen, and Carmichael (1992).

14. Stephan and Andy (1970).

15. Descriptions of the connections between these areas and other cortical regions may be found in Van Hoesen (1982); Van Hoesen and Pandya (1975); and Van Hoesen, Pandya, and Butters (1972, 1975). The existence of stable, widespread ensembles with preferential connections would not in itself be enough to create integrated perceptual experience or recall. Other brain circuits may be responsible for producing perceptual unity by temporally coordinating the neural activity that represents component features of the sensory world (see, for example, Sillito, Jones, Gerstein, and West, 1994).

16. Recanzone, Schreiner, and Merzenich (1993).

17. Weinberger (1993).

18. Neuropathological findings, and discussions regarding the involvement of the amygdala and other structures in autism, may be found in Courchesne (1991); Piven et al. (1990); Bauman and Kemper (1985, 1988, 1994); and Fein, Pennington, and Waterhouse (1987).

19. These studies are documented in Bachevalier (1991), and Bachevalier and Merjanian (1994).

20. Studies summarized in this section are from Asberg, Thoren, and Traskman (1976); Asberg, Traskman, and Thoren (1976); Brown, Goodwin, Ballenger, Goyer, and Major (1979); Kruesi et al. (1990); Linnoila et al. (1983); Higley et al. (1992); Raleigh et al. (1986); Raleigh et al. (1980); and Mehlman et al. (1995).

21. Raleigh, McGuire, Brammer, Pollack, and Yuwiler (1991).

22. Raleigh and Brammer (1993).

CHAPTER 5

1. Rorty (1979).

2. Kling et al. (1992).

3. See Shapin and Schaffer (1985) and Shapin (1994) for historical accounts of the practices and arguments through which experimental science established itself as a purely objective enterprise.

4. The aspects of prosopagnosia reviewed here are discussed in more detail in Damasio, Tranel, and Damasio (1990a) and Damasio (1989a).

5. Heywood and Cowie (1992).

6. The articles referred to in this section are by Desimone, Albright, Gross, and Bruce (1984); Desimone (1991); Gross (1992); Gross and Sergeant (1992); and Kendrick and Baldwin (1987).

7. Conversations with Alan Bond, Isabel Gauthier, and Valerie Stone on this issue were helpful.

8. Delgado (1967, pp. 177, 186).

9. Grant and Redmond (1984, p. 707).

10. Hamburg (1963); Tooby and DeVore (1987).

11. See Révész (1956). Regarding imitation in apes and monkeys, see De-Waal (1982) and Hauser (1988). Révész pointed out that feelings of belonging establish and stabilize communities; it is only in a stable community that collective purposes can be realized through the joint activity of members.

12. Excerpt from Le Bon (1903, pp. 29, 46).

13. Excerpt from Kerckhoff and Back (1968, pp. 39–40). The term "hysterical contagion" is used on p.12.

14. R. Barton, personal communication, June 15, 1990.

15. The preceding studies are found in Pawlby (1977); Meltzoff (1990); Uzgiris, Benson, Kruper, and Vasek (1989); Meltzoff and Gopnik (1993); Bretherton (1992); Scaife and Bruner (1975); and Nelson and Seidman (1984).

16. It is usually believed that there is a capacity called empathy that is a kind of knowing in which the object of knowledge is another mind. But the independent reality of the other mind has to be assumed in order for empathy to be like mind reading rather than mind making; my purpose in this book is to show that minds are *made*—by other brains. They are made, not read or known as one would read or know external signs and objects.

Furthermore, it's not possible to establish whether two subjectivities "know" one another except by the assent of the "knowee." This cannot constitute independent proof of knowing, just as assent to an interpretation of unconscious motive cannot constitute proof of the operation of that motive (as pointed out by Bouveresse, 1995). We must conclude that intersubjective "understanding" is simply a state of affairs in which parties signal to one another that the state has been achieved.

17. The sociologist Herbert Blumer wrote about the loss of self-consciousness in the setting of social contagion. Normal self-consciousness, he wrote, "is a means of barricading oneself against the influence of others." (Blumer, 1939, p. 176).

18. Rizzolatti, Fadiga, Gallese, and Fogassi (1996); Gallese, Fadiga, Fogassi, and Rizzolatti (1996).

CHAPTER 6

1. "When someone tells you a story in response to one you have told that captures an important generalization between the two, you believe that you have been 'really understood' and you ascribe qualities of high intelligence and perception to your listener." "Storytelling and understanding are functionally the same thing" (Schank, 1990, pp. 21, 24).

2. Narration can be thought of as the description of actions, in which actions are performed by persons, keeping in mind that any telling presents only one version out of the many versions that are possible. Bruner's approach tends in the direction of seeing narrative as rhetorical or justificatory in function, and also recognizes the centrality of persons and their actions as the subject matter of narrative (Bruner, 1990). Schafer's (1992) approach, in

contrast, characterizes not only the subject matter of narrative, but also its formal elements.

3. Excerpt from pp. 225–226 of Goodwin, C. (1984). Notes on story structure and the organization of participation. In M. Atkinson and J. Heritage (Eds.), *Structures of Social Action: Studies in Conversation Analysis* (pp. 225–246). Cambridge: Cambridge University Press. © Maison de Sciences de l'Homme and Cambridge University Press 1984. Reprinted with the permission of Cambridge University Press.

4. For discussion of memes, see Dennett (1991, p. 200). A 2-year-old's reenvoicements are described in Dore (1989).

5. Bruner and Feldman (1993).

6. For a detailed philosophical discussion of the relations between reasons and causes, see Davidson (1980).

7. Sacks (1984).

8. From Harré (1984, p. 65).

9. Eliot (1871–1872/1988, p. 615).

10. Excerpt from Patry and Nespoulous (1990, p. 20).

11. See Perinbanayagam (1991).

12. Goosen (1987); Dunbar (1993).

13. Sacks, Schegloff, and Jefferson (1974); Leiter (1980, p. 216).

14. Excerpt from p. 239 of Goodwin, C. (1984). Notes on story structure and the organization of participation. In M. Atkinson and J. Heritage (Eds.), *Structures of social action: studies in conversation Analysis*. Cambridge: Cambridge University Press, pp. 225–246. Copyright © Maison de Sciences de l'Homme and Cambridge University Press 1984. Reprinted with the permission of Cambridge University Press.

15. Bavelas and Chovil (1995).

16. Excerpt from Rinn (1984, p. 56).

17. Excerpt from p. 183 of Ekman, P. (1979). About brows: Emotional and conversational signals. In J. Aschoof, M. von Cranach, K. Foppa, W. Lepenies, D. Ploog (Eds.), *Human Ethology: Claims and Limits of a New Discipline*. Cambridge: Cambridge University Press, pp. 169–202. Copyright © Cambridge University Press 1979. Reprinted by permission of Cambridge University Press.

18. Ekman (1979).

19. Chovil (1989).

20. From Allman, J., and McGuinness, E. (1988, p. 282). Visual cortex in primates. In *Comparative Primate Biology, vol. 4: Neurosciences*. New York: Alan R. Liss, pp. 279–326. Copyright © Alan R. Liss, 1986. Reprinted by permission of John Wiley and Sons, Inc.

21. Rinn (1984, p. 58).

22. Darwin (1872/1965, p. 364.)

23. Gazzaniga and Smylie (1990).

24. Ekman and Friesen (1982).

25. Provine (1993).

26. Fry (1977).

27. The role of prefrontal cortex in the temporal organization of behavior has been studied by Fuster and is reviewed in Fuster (1989). Face-responsive neurons in monkey prefrontal areas are described in Pigarev, Rizzolatti, and Scandolara (1979) and in Wilson, Ó Scalaidhe and Goldman-Rakic (1993). Conversational problems following frontal lobe lesions are reported by Alexander, Benson, and Stuss (1989).

28. Darwin (1872/1965, pp. 48–49).

CHAPTER 7

1. Readers already familiar with Mead will note his influence throughout much of this book. The works referred to in succeeding paragraphs are Mead (1934); Wittgenstein (1953); Wertsch (1985); Harré (1984); Dennett (1991); and James (1890). James' discussion of the self is found on p. 337. His term "common-sense" deserves particular attention, because it is thought held *in common* that is at issue in social constructionism.

2. Excerpt from Mead, G.H. (1934). *Mind, self and society from the standpoint of a social behaviorist* (pp. 161–162). Chicago: The University of Chicago Press. Copyright © 1962, The University of Chicago.

3. Regarding the relation between Mead's work and that of Wittgenstein, see Miller (1973, pp. 67, 74).

4. Excerpt from Harré (1984, pp. 145–146).

5. Theories and findings on sensory awareness based on the physiology of individual brains include, for example, Crick and Koch, (1990, 1995) and Kolb and Braun (1995). The following have put forward views of consciousness that are socially based, as well as biologically oriented: Trevarthen (1979); Trevarthen and Logotheti (1989); Crook (1988); and Humphrey (1984). Although Trevarthen shows that aspects of awareness are affected by interruption of interhemispheric connections, theorists emphasizing the social functions of consciousness generally provide little detail regarding its neural basis.

6. Excerpts in this section are from Keller (1954, pp. 36, 37, 256, 257).

7. Regarding the composition of signs of the self, see Singer (1980); Perinbanayagam (1990); and Battershill (1990). For a synopsis of Mead's views on individual creativity, see Miller's (1973) chapter on creativity.

8. Ethnomethodological studies in this section are reported in Leiter (1974, 1976); Wieder (1974); and Garfinkel (1967). For an overview of ethnomethodology see Heritage (1984). Excerpt is from Wieder, 1974 (pp. 203–204).

9. See Schutz (1962, pp. 11–12).

10. Dilthey (1989, p. 61).

11. Stent (1975, p. 1057).

12. See Churchland, P. (1986, p. 343).

13. For a simulation of primate brain function that embeds brains in social groups, see Bond (1996) and http://www.vision.caltech.edu/bond.

CHAPTER 8

1. Ekman (1977, pp. 61–62).

2. Excerpt from p. 1057 of LeDoux (1995). In search of an emotional system in the brain: Leaping from fear to emotion and consciousness. In M. Gazzaniga, (Ed.), *The Cognitive Neurosciences* (pp. 1049–1061). Cambridge, MA: MIT Press. © 1995 Massachusetts Institute of Technology.

3. LeDoux (1991).

4. From Broca (1888, p. 260); Papez (1937); and MacLean (1952).

5. From LeDoux (1991, p.190).

6. Dennett (1991).

7. Kling stated that the pattern of inputs and outputs that couples high-level sensory representations directly with effector activity "*is* emotion." See Kling and Brothers (1992). For a detailed analysis of inputs and outputs of the amygdala and other structures along these lines, see Brothers (1995).

8. Damasio (1994).

9. Ekman and Friesen (1982, p. 239).

10. Excerpt from p. 96 of Fridlund, A. (1992). The behavioral ecology and sociality of human faces. In M. Clark., (Ed.), *Emotion*. Newbury Park: Sage, pp. 90–121. Copyright © 1992 by Sage Publications, Inc. Reprinted by permission of Sage Publications, Inc.

11. The social-context-based accounts reviewed here are from Fridlund (1991a, 1991b, 1992); Karakashian, Gyger, and Marler (1988); Kraut and Johnston (1979); and Chovil (1991). For discussion of some of these studies, see Buck (1991).

12. Ekman and Friesen (1969); Buck (1991).

13. Regarding "basic" emotions, see Panksepp (1982); Ekman (1992); and Ortony and Turner (1990).

14. Etcoff and Magee (1992).

15. Kemper (1987); Hochschild (1979).

16. Coulter (1989, p. 43); Perinbanayagam (1991, pp. 145, 148).

17. From Izard and Haynes (1988, p.14).

18. Stern (1985).

19. My discussion here echoes that of Bruner (1990, pp. 13–15). Because, as E. Doyle McCarthy points out, we live in "an age of psychological and therapeutic knowledge and practice," the institutions and social relations of our world dictate that emotions shall exist and have significance (McCarthy, 1989, p. 66).

CHAPTER 9

1. This distinction is pointed out in Bouveresse (1995).

2. Schafer (1992); Spence (1982). The excerpts are from Spence (1982, pp. 35–36, p. 284). Schafer's (1992) account of the response to an interpretation is found on page 182.

3. Excerpt from Schafer, R. (1992). *Retelling a Life: Narration and Dialogue in Psychoanalysis* (p.xv). New York: Basic Books. Copyright © 1992 Basic Books, a division of HarperCollins Publishers, Inc. Reprinted with permission.

4. See Sullivan (1953). "Two-body" psychoanalysis began with Balint and Balint (1939) and Balint (1949/1965). For reviews see Greenberg and Mitchell (1983) and Bacal and Newman (1990).

5. Reprinted from Robert D. Stolorow and George E. Atwood, *Contexts of Being: The Intersubjective Foundations of Psychological Life* (Hillsdale, N.J.: The Analytic Press, 1992), pp. 121–122 by permission. Copyright © 1992 by The Analytic Press.

6. Much relevant acculturation precedes the clinical encounter, making the encounter itself intelligible to the patient. The preceding acculturation is provided by the larger society, which already subscribes to the vocabulary of the unconscious and other metapsychological concepts. Burke pointed this out long ago. One is constrained to explain one's motives to oneself using the vocabulary of motives current in one's group, thus, "A generally accepted account as to how the mind works can make the mind work that way." (Burke, 1935, p. 43)

7. From Harré (1984, p. 65).

8. Greenson (1971/1978, pp. 415–423).

9. From Bollas (1989, p. 108).

10. Hobson (1992).

11. From Bruner (1990, p. 60).

12. Excerpts from pp. 236, 238 of Schwaber, E. (1990) Interpretation and the therapeutic action of psychoanalysis, *International Journal of Psychoanalysis*. 71, 229–240. Copyright © Institute of Psychoanalysis. Reprinted with permission.

13. Excerpted from Perinbanayagam (1990, p. 317). (A typographical omission in the original passage is corrected here.)

14. Excerpt from Bion (1967, pp. 272, 273). "Notes on Memory and Desire" by Wilfred R. Bion, M.D. was first published in *The Psychoanalytic Forum*, Volume 2, number 3, Autumn 1967, John A. Lindon, M.D., Editor. Copyright © The Psychiatric Research Foundation. Reprinted with permission.

15. Excerpts from pp. 165, 167–168 of Fierman, L. (Ed.) (1965). *Effective Psychotherapy: The Contribution of Hellmuth Kaiser*. New York: The Free Press. Copyright © 1969 by The Free Press, a division of Simon and Schuster, Inc. Reprinted with permission of the publisher.

CHAPTER 10

1. The mingling of everyday and scientific explanation is very characteristic of much of the speculative writing that attempts to explain psychology in terms of biology. This genre usually has a gauche, pseudoscientific quality.

Occasionally, though, the underlying confusion produces a well-told tale, and the hybrid is quite charming. For example, Freud's (1900) *The Interpretation of Dreams* confuses reasons and causes — but it comes across less as bad science than as a good story, whose characters (Pcs., Ucs., the sleeper, the instincts) struggle and compromise, reveal and deceive.

    2. Excerpted from Malcolm (1986, p. 200).

References

Adolphs, R., Tranel, D., Damasio, H., and Damasio, A. (1994). Impaired recognition of emotion in facial expressions following bilateral damage to the human amygdala. *Nature, 372,* 669–672.

Adolphs, R., Tranel, D., Damasio, H., and Damasio, A. (1995). Fear and the human amygdala. *Journal of Neuroscience, 15,* 5879–5891.

Alexander, M., Benson, D., and Stuss, D. (1989). Frontal lobes and language. *Brain and Language, 37,* 656–691.

Allman, J., and McGuinness, E. (1988). Visual cortex in primates. In *Comparative primate biology, vol. 4: Neurosciences* (pp. 279–326). New York: Alan R. Liss.

Amaral, D., Price, J.L., Pitkanen, A., and Carmichael, S.T. (1992). Anatomical organization of the primate amygdaloid complex. In J. P. Aggleton (Ed.), *The Amygdala: Neurobiological aspects of emotion, memory, and mental dysfunction* (pp. 1–66). New York: Wiley-Liss.

Ardila, A., Botero, M., Gomez, J., and Quijano, C. (1988). Partial cognitive-dysmnesic seizures as a model for studying psychosis. *International Journal Neuroscience, 38,* 11–20.

Ardila, A., and Rosseli, M. (1988). Temporal lobe involvement in Capgras syndrome. *International Journal Neuroscience, 43,* 219–224.

Aronson, E., and Rosenbloom, S. (1971). Space perception in early infancy: Perception within a common auditory-visual space. *Science, 172,* 1161–1163.

Asberg, M., Thoren, P., and Traskman, L. (1976). "Serotonin depression"—A biochemical subgroup within the affective disorders? *Science, 191,* 478–480.

Asberg, M., Traskman, L., and Thoren, P. (1976). 5-HIAA in the cerebrospinal fluid: A biochemical suicide predictor? *Archives of Gen. Psychiatry, 33,* 1193–1197.

Attwood, A., Frith, U., and Hermelin, B. (1988). The understanding and use of interpersonal gestures by autistic and Down's syndrome children. *Journal of Autism and Developmental Disorders, 18*: 241–257.

Ayer, A. (1963). The concept of a person and other essays. New York: St. Martin's Press Inc.

Bacal, H., and Newman, K. (1990). Theories of object relations: Bridges to self psychology. New York: Columbia University Press.

Bachevalier, J. (1991). An animal model for childhood autism: Memory loss and socioemotional disturbances following neonatal damage to the limbic system in monkeys. In C.A. Tamminga and S.C. Schulz (Eds.), *Advances in neuropsychiatry and psychopharmacology, Vol. 1, schizophrenia research* (pp. 129–140). New York: Raven Press.

Bachevalier J., and Merjanian, P. (1994). The contribution of medial temporal lobe structures in infantile autism: A neurobehavioral study in primates. In M. Bauman (Ed.), *The Neurobiology of Autism* (pp. 146–169). Baltimore: Johns Hopkins University Press.

Baizer, J.S., Ungerleider, L.G., and Desimone, R. (1991). Organization of visual inputs to the inferior temporal and posterior parietal cortex in macaques. *Journal of Neuroscience, 11*, 168–190.

Balint, M. (1965). Changing therapeutical aims and techniques in psychoanalysis. In *Primary love and psycho-analytic technique* (pp. 209–222). London, Butler and Tanner (Original work published 1949).

Balint, M., and Balint, A. (1939). On transference and counter-transference, *International Journal of Psychoanalysis, 20*, 223–230.

Barlow, H. (1953). Summation and inhibition in the frog's retina. *Journal of Physiology, 119*, 69–88.

Barlow, H., Fitzhigh, R., and Kuffler, S. (1957). Change of organization in the receptive fields of the cat's retina during dark adaptation. *Journal of Physiology, 137*, 338–354.

Baron-Cohen, S. (1988). Social and pragmatic deficits in autism: Cognitive or affective? *Journal of Autism and Developmental Disorders, 18*, 379–402.

Baron-Cohen, S. (1989). Perceptual roletaking and protodeclarative pointing in autism. *British Journal of Developmental Psychology, 7*, 113–127.

Baron-Cohen, S. (1992). The theory of mind hypothesis of autism: History and prospects of the idea. *Psychologist, 5*, 9–12.

Baron-Cohen, S. (1995). *Mindblindness*. Cambridge: MIT Press.

Baron-Cohen, S., and Cross, P. (1992). Reading the eyes: Evidence for the role of perception in the development of a theory of mind. *Mind and Language, 6*, 173–186.

Baron-Cohen, S., and Ring, H. (1994). A model of the mind-reading system: Neuropsychological and neurobiological perspectives. In P. Mitchell, and C. Lewis (Eds.), *Origins of an Understanding of Mind* (pp. 183–207). Hillsdale, NJ: Lawrence Erlbaum.

Battershill, C. (1990). Erving Goffman as a precursor to post-modern sociology. In S. Riggins (Ed.), *Beyond Goffman: Studies on Communication, Insti-*

tution, and Social Interaction (pp.163–186). New York: Mouton de Gruyter.

Bauman, M., and Kemper, T. (1985). Histoanatomic observations of the brain in early infantile autism. *Neurology, 35*, 866–874.

Bauman, M., and Kemper, T. (1988). Limbic and cerebellar abnormalities: Consistent findings in infantile autism. *Journal of Neuropathology and Experimental Neurophysiology, 47*, 369.

Bauman, M., and Kemper, T. (1994). Neuroanatomic observations of the brain in autism. In M. Bauman (Ed.), *The Neurobiology of Autism* (pp. 119–145). Baltimore: Johns Hopkins University Press.

Bavelas, J., and Chovil, N. (1995). An integrated message model of language in face-to-face dialogue. Manuscript submitted for publication.

Baylis, G., Rolls, E.T., and Leonard, C.M. (1985). Selectivity between faces in the responses of a population of neurons in the cortex in the superior temporal sulcus of the monkey. *Brain Research, 342*, 91–102.

Bion, W. (1967). Notes on memory and desire. *Psychoanalytic Forum, 2*, 272–273.

Blumer, H. (1939). Collective behavior. In A. Lee (Ed.), *Principles of Sociology* (pp. 165–222). New York: Barnes and Noble.

Bollas, C. (1989). *Forces of destiny: Psychoanalysis and the human idiom.* London: Free Association Books.

Bond, A. (1996). A Computational architecture for social agents. In *Proceedings of Intelligent Systems: A Semiotic Perspective, An International Multidisciplinary Conference*, National Institute of Standards and Technolgy.

Boussaoud, D., Ungerleider, L.G., and Desimone, R. (1990). Pathways for motion analysis: Cortical connections of the medial superior temporal and fundus of the superior temporal visual areas in the macaque. *Journal of Comparative Neurology, 296*, 462–495.

Bouveresse, J. (1995). *Wittgenstein reads Freud: The myth of the unconscious.* Princeton, NJ: Princeton University Press.

Bretherton, I. (1992). Social referencing, intentional communication, and the interfacing of minds in infancy. In S. Feinman (Ed.), *Social Referencing and the Social Construction of Reality in Infancy* (pp.57–77). New York: Plenum Press.

Broca, P. (1888). *Memoires sur le cerveau de l'Homme et des primates.* [Reports on the brain of man and primates] Paris: C. Reinwald, Editeur.

Brothers, L. (1990). The social brain: a project for integrating primate behavior and neurophysiology in a new domain. *Concepts in Neuroscience, 1*, 27–51.

Brothers, L. (1994). Socialization, communication and imagination. *Cahiers de Psychologie Cognitive, 13*, 561–564.

Brothers, L. (1995). Neurophysiology of the perception of intentions by primates. In M. Gazzaniga (Ed.), *The Cognitive Neurosciences* (pp. 1107–1115).Cambridge: MIT Press.

Brothers, L., and Ring, B. (1992). A neuroethological framework for the representation of minds. *Journal of Cognitive Neuroscience, 4*, 107–118.

Brothers, L., and Ring, B. (1993). Mesial temporal neurons in the macaque monkey with responses selective for aspects of social stimuli. *Behavioural Brain Research, 57*, 53–61.

Brothers, L., Ring, B., and Kling, A.S. (1990). Response of neurons in the macaque amygdala to complex social stimuli. *Behavioural Brain Research, 41*, 199–213.

Brown, G., and Goodwin, F., Ballenger, J., Goyer, P., and Major, L. (1979). Aggression in humans correlates with cerebrospinal fluid amine metabolites. *Psychiatry Research, 1*, 131–139.

Brown S., and Schäfer, E.A. (1888). An investigation into the functions of the occipital and temporal lobes of the monkey's brain. *Philosophical Transactions of the Royal Society of London, 179*, 303–327.

Bruce, C., Desimone, R., and Gross, C.G. (1981). Visual properties of neurons in a polysensory area in superior temporal sulcus of the macaque. *Journal Neurophysiology, 46*, 369–384.

Bruce, V. (1988). *Recognizing faces.* East Sussex, UK: Lawrence Erlbaum.

Bruner, J. (1990). *Acts of meaning.* Cambridge, MA: Harvard University Press.

Bruner, J., and Feldman, C. (1993). Theories of mind and the problem of autism. In S. Baron-Cohen, H. Tager-Flusberg, and D. Cohen (Eds.), *Understanding Other Minds: Perspectives from Autism* (pp. 267–291). Oxford: Oxford University Press.

Burke, K. (1935). *Permanence and change: An anatomy of purpose.* New York: New Republic.

Buck, R. (1991). Social factors in facial display and communication: A reply to Chovil and others. *Journal of Nonverbal Behavior, 15*: 155–161.

Campbell, R. (1992). The neuropsychology of lipreading. *Philosophical Transactions of the Royal Society of London Series B, 335*, 39–45.

Campbell, R., Garwood, J., Franklin, S., Howard, D., Landis, T., and Regard, M. (1990). Neuropsychological studies of auditory-visual fusion illusions. Four case studies and their implications. *Neuropsychologia, 28*, 787–802.

Campbell, R., Landis, T., and Regard, M. (1986). Face recognition and lipreading: A neurological dissociation. *Brain, 109*, 509–521.

Charman, T., and Baron-Cohen, S. (1995). Understanding photos, models, and beliefs: A test of the modularity thesis of theory of mind. *Cognitive Development, 10*, 287–298.

Cheney, D., and Seyfarth, R. (1990). *How monkeys see the world: Inside the mind of another species.* Chicago: University of Chicago Press.

Cheney, D., Seyfarth, R., and Smuts, B. (1986). Social relationships and social cognition in nonhuman primates. *Science, 234*, 1361–1366.

Chovil, N. (1989). *Communicative Functions of Facial Displays in Conversation,* Unpublished doctoral dissertation, University of Victoria, Canada.

Chovil, N. (1991). Social determinants of facial displays. *Journal of Nonverbal Behavior, 15*, 141–154.

Churchland, P. (1986). *Neurophilosophy: Toward a unified science of the mind/brain*. Cambridge, MA: MIT Press.

Cicone, M., Wapner, W., and Gardner, H. (1980). Sensitivity to emotional expressions and situations in organic patients. *Cortex, 16,* 145–158.

Corina, D., Vaid, J., and Bellugi, U. (1992). The linguistic basis of left hemisphere specialization, *Science, 255,* 1258–1260.

Coulter, J. (1989). Cognitive "penetrability" and the emotions. In D. Franks and E. McCarthy (Eds.), *The Sociology of Emotions: Original Essays and Research Papers* (pp. 33–50). Greenwich, CT: JAI Press, Inc.

Courchesne, E. (1987). A neurophysiological view of autism. In E. Schopler, G. Mesibov (Eds.), *Neurobiological Issues in Autism* (pp. 285–324). New York: Plenum Press.

Courchesne, E. (1991). Neuroanatomic imaging in autism. *Pediatrics, 87,* (pt.2), 781–790.

Crick, F., and Koch, C. (1990). Towards a neurobiological theory of consciousness. *Seminars in Neuroscience, 2,* 263–275.

Crick, F., and Koch, C. (1995). Are we aware of neural activity in primary visual cortex? *Nature, 375,* 121–123.

Crook, J. (1988). The experiential context of intellect. In R. Byrne, A. Whiten (Eds.), *Machiavellian Intelligence: Social Expertise and the Evolution of Intellect in Monkeys, Apes, and Humans* (pp. 347–362). Oxford: Clarendon Press.

Damasio, A. (1989a). Reflections on visual recogition. In A. Galaburda (Ed.), *From reading to Neurons* (pp. 361–376). Cambridge, MA: MIT Press.

Damasio, A. (1989b). The brain binds entities and events by multiregional activation from convergence zones. *Neural Computation, 1,* 123–132.

Damasio, A. (1994). *Descartes' error: Emotion, reason, and the human brain.* New York: G.P. Putnam's Sons.

Damasio, A., Tranel, D., and Damasio, H. (1990a). Face agnosia and the neural substrates of memory. *Annual Review of Neuroscience, 13,* 89–109.

Damasio, A., Tranel, D., and Damasio, H., (1990b). Individuals with sociopathic behavior caused by frontal damage fail to respond autonomically to social stimuli. *Behavioural Brain Research, 41,* 81–94.

Damasio, A., and van Hoesen, G. (1983). Emotional disturbances associated with focal lesions of the limbic frontal lobe. In K. Heilman, P. Satz (Eds.), *Neuropsychology of human emotion* (pp.85–110). New York: Guilford Press.

Darwin, C. (1965). *The expression of the emotions in man and animals.* Chicago: The University of Chicago Press. (Original work published 1872.)

Davidson, D. (1980). *Essays on actions and events.* Oxford: Clarendon Press.

Defoe, D. (1957). *Robinson Crusoe.* New York: Charles Scribner's Sons. (Original work published 1719.)

Delgado, J.M.R. (1967). Aggression and defense under cerebral radio control. In C. Clemente, D. Lindsley (Eds.), *Aggression and Defense: Neural Mecha-*

nisms and Social Patterns, Proceedings of the Fifth Conference on Brain Function (pp. 171–193). Berkeley, CA: University of California Press.

Dennett, D. (1991). *Consciousness explained.* Boston: Little, Brown.

Desimone, R. (1991). Face-selective cells in the temporal cortex of monkeys. *Journal of Cognitive Neuroscience, 3,* 1–8.

Desimone, R., Albright, T., Gross, C., and Bruce, C. (1984). Stimulus-selective properties of inferior temporal neurons in the macaque. *Journal of Neuroscience, 4,* 2051–2062.

DeWaal, F. (1982). *Chimpanzee politics.* Baltimore: Johns Hopkins University Press.

Dicks, D., Myers, R., and Kling, A.S. (1969). Uncus and amygdala lesions: Effects on social behavior in the free-ranging rhesus monkey. *Science, 165,* 69–71.

Dilthey, W. (1989). *Selected Works, Vol 1: Introduction to the Human Sciences.* Makkreel, R., Rodi, F. (Eds.), Princeton, NJ: Princeton University Press.

Dore, J. (1989). Monologue as reenvoicement of dialogue. In K. Nelson (Ed.), *Narratives from the Crib* (pp. 231–260). Cambridge, MA: Harvard University Press.

Douglas, M. (1992). The person in an enterprise culture. In S.H. Heap and A. Ross (Eds.), *Understanding the Enterprise Culture: Themes in the Work of Mary Douglas* (pp. 41–62). Edinburgh: Edinburgh University Press.

Downer, J. (1962). Interhemispheric integration in the visual system. In V. Mountcastle (Ed.), *Interhemispheric Relations and Cerebral Dominance* (pp. 87–100). Baltimore: The Johns Hopkins Press.

Dunbar, R. (1993). Coevolution of neocortical size, group size and language in humans. *Behavioral and Brain Sci*ences, *16,* 681–735.

Eichenbaum, H. (1993). Thinking about brain cell assemblies. *Science, 26,* 993–94.

Ekman, P. (1977). Biological and cultural contributions to body and facial movement. In J. Blacking (Ed.), *Anthropology of the Body* (pp. 34–84). San Diego: Academic Press.

Ekman, P. (1979). About brows: Emotional and conversational signals. In J. Aschoof, M. von Cranach, K. Foppa, W. Lepenies, D. Ploog (Eds.), *Human Ethology: Claims and Limits of a New Discipline* (pp. 169–202). Cambridge, UK: Cambridge University Press.

Ekman, P. (1992). Are there basic emotions? *Psychological Revi*ew, *99,* 550–553.

Ekman, P., and Friesen, W. (1969). The repertoire of nonverbal behavior—Categories, origins, usage, and coding. *Semiotica, 1,* 49–98.

Ekman, P., and Friesen, W. (1982). Felt, false and miserable smiles. *Journal of Nonverbal Behavior, 6,* 238–252.

Eliot, G. (1988). *Middlemarch.* New York: Oxford University Press. (Original work published 1871–1872)

Ellis, H., de Pauw, K., Christodoulou, G., Papageorgiou, L., Milne, A., Joseph, A. (1993). Responses to facial and non-facial stimuli presented tachistoscopically in either or both visual fields by patients with the Capgras delusion and paranoid schizophrenics. *Journal of Neurology, Neurosurgery and Psychiatry, 56,* 215–219.

Eslinger, P.J., and Damasio, A. (1985). Severe disturbance of higher cognition after bilateral frontal lobe ablations: Patient EVR. *Neurology, 35,* 1731–1741.

Etcoff, N., and Magee, J. (1992). Categorical perception of facial expressions. *Cognition, 44,* 227–240.

Fay, W. (1979). Personal pronouns and the autistic child. *Journal of Autism and Developmental Disorders, 9,* 247–260.

Fein, D., Pennington, B., and Waterhouse, L. (1987). Implications of social deficits in autism for neurological dysfunction. In E. Schopler, G. Mesibov (Eds.), *Neurobiological Issues in Autism* (pp. 127–144). New York: Plenum.

Feinberg, T., and Shapiro, R. (1989). Misidentification-reduplication and the right hemisphere. *Neuropsychiatry, Neuropsychology, and Behavioral Neurology, 2,* 39–48.

Fernald, A., Taeschner, T., Dunn, J., Papousek, M., de Boysson-Bardies, B., and Fukui, I. (1989). A cross-language study of prosodic modifications in mothers' and fathers' speech to preverbal infants. *Journal of Child Language, 16,* 477–501.

Field, T., Woodson, R., Greenberg, R., and Cohen, D. (1982). Discrimination and imitation of facial expression by neonates. *Science, 218,* 179–181.

Fierman, L., Ed. (1965). *Effective psychotherapy: The contribution of Hellmuth Kaiser.* New York: Free Press.

Fodor, J. (1992). Discussion: A theory of the child's theory of mind. *Cognition, 44,* 283–296.

Freud, S. (1900). The interpretation of dreams. In J. Strachey (Ed. and Trans.), *The standard edition of the complete psychological works* (3d ed., vols 4, 5). London: Hogarth Press.

Fridlund, A. (1991a). Evolution and facial action in reflex, social motive, and paralanguage. *Biological Psychology, 32,* 3–100.

Fridlund, A. (1991b). The sociality of solitary smiling: Potentiation by an implicit audience. *Journal of Personality and Social Psychology, 60,* 229–240.

Fridlund, A. (1992). The behavioral ecology and sociality of human faces. In M. Clark (Ed.), *Emotion* (pp. 90–121). Newbury Park,CA: Sage.

Fried, I., Mateer, C., Ojemann, G., Wohns, R., and Fedio, P. (1982). Organization of visuospatial functions in human cortex. *Brain, 105,* 349–371.

Frith, U. (1989). *Autism: Explaining the enigma.* Oxford, UK: Blackwell.

Fry, D. (1977). *Homo loquens: Man as a talking animal.* London: Cambridge University Press.

Fuster, J. (1989). *The prefrontal cortex: Anatomy, physiology, and neuropsychology of the frontal lobes* (2nd Ed.). New York: Raven Press.

Gallese, V., Fadiga, L., Fogassi, L., and Rizzolatti G., (1996). Action recognition in the premotor cortex. *Brain, 119,* 593–609.

Garfinkel, H. (1967). *Studies in Ethnomethodology* (pp. 116–185). Englewood Cliffs, NJ: Prentice-Hall.

Gazzaniga, M., and Smylie, C. (1990). Hemispheric mechanisms controlling voluntary and spontaneous facial expressions. *Journal of Cognitive Neuroscience 2*, 239–245.

Gerber, E.R. (1985). Rage and obligation: Samoan emotion in conflict. In G.M. White, J. Kirkpatrick (Eds.), *Person, Self, and Experience: Exploring Pacific Ethnopsychologies* (pp. 121–167). Los Angeles: University of California Press.

Gloor, P. (1986) The role of the human limbic system in perception, memory and affect: Lessons from temporal lobe epilepsy. In B.K. Doane, K.E. Livingston (Eds.), *The Limbic System: Functional Organization and Clinical Disorders* (pp. 159–169). New York: Raven Press.

Gloor, P. (1990). Experiential phenomena of temporal lobe epilepsy: Facts and hypotheses. *Brain, 113*, 1673–1694.

Goffman, E. (1967). *Interaction ritual: Essays on face-to-face behavior*. Garden City, NY: Anchor Books.

Goffman, E. (1974). *Frame analysis: An essay on the organization of experience*. Cambridge, MA: Harvard University Press.

Goodwin, C. (1984). Notes on story structure and the organization of participation. In M. Atkinson, J. Heritage (Eds.), *Structures of social action: Studies in conversation analysis* (pp. 225–246). Cambridge.UK: Cambridge University Press.

Goosen, C. (1987). Social grooming in primates. *Comparative Primate Biology, Vol 2B: Behavior, Cognition and Motivation*, 107–131.

Goren, C., Sarty, M., and Wu, P. (1975). Visual following and pattern discrimination of face-like stimuli by newborn infants. *Pediatrics, 56*, 544–549.

Grant, S., and Redmond, D. (1984). Neuronal activity of the locus coeruleus in awake *Macaca arctoides*. *Experimental Neurology, 84*, 701–709.

Greenberg, J., and Mitchell, S., (1983). Interpersonal psychoanalysis. In *Object relations in psychoanalytic theory*. Cambridge, MA: Harvard University Press.

Greenson, R. (1978). *Explorations in Psychoanalysis* (pp. 415–423). New York: International Universities Press. (Original work published 1971.)

Gross, C. (1992). Representation of visual stimuli in inferior temporal cortex. *Philosophical Transactions of the Royal Society of London Series B, 335*, 3–10.

Gross, C., Bender, D., and Rocha-Miranda, C. (1969). Visual receptive fields of neurons in inferotemporal cortex of the monkey. *Science, 166*, 1303–1306.

Gross, C., Rocha-Miranda, C., and Bender, D. (1972). Visual properties of neurons in inferotemporal cortex of the macaque. *Journal of Neurophysiology, 35*, 96–111.

Gross, C., and Sergeant, J. (1992). Face recognition. *Current Opinion in Neurobiology, 2*, 156–161.

Haith, M., Bergman, T., and Moore, M. (1977). Eye contact and face scanning in early infancy. *Science, 198,* 853–855.

Hamann, S., Stefanacci, L., Squire, L., Adolphs, R., Tranel, D., Damasio, H., and Damasio, A. (1996). Recognizing facial emotion. *Nature, 379,* 497.

Hamburg, D.A. (1963). Emotions in the perspective of human evolution. In P.E. Knapp, (Ed.), *Expression of the emotions in man* (pp. 300–317). New York: International Universities Press.

Harré, R. (1984). *Personal being: A theory for individual psychology.* Cambridge,MA: Harvard University Press.

Harré, R. (1993). *Social being* (2nd ed.). Oxford: Blackwell.

Hasselmo, M.E., Rolls, E.T., and Baylis, G.C. (1989). The role of expression and identity in the face-selective responses of neurons in the temporal visual cortex of the monkey. *Behavioral Brain Research, 32,* 203–218.

Hauser, M. (1988). Invention and social transmission: New data from wild vervet monkeys. In R. Byrne, A. Whiten (Eds.), *Machiavellian intelligence: Social expertise and the evolution of intellect in monkeys, apes, and humans* (pp. 327–343). Oxford, UK: Clarendon Press.

Heritage, J. (1984). *Garfinkel and ethnomethodology.* Cambridge,UK: Polity.

Heywood, C., and Cowey, A. (1992). The role of the "face-cell" area in the discrimination and recognition of faces by monkeys. *Philosophical Transactions of the Royal Society of London Series B, 335,* 31–38.

Higley, J., Mehlman, P., Taub, D., Higley, S., Suomi, S., Linnoila, M., and Vickers, J. (1992). Cerebrospinal fluid monoamine and adrenal correlates of aggression in free-ranging rhesus monkeys. *Archives of General Psychiatry, 49,* 436–44.

Hobson, J. (1992). The brain as a dream machine: An activation-synthesis hypothesis of dreaming. In M. Lansky (Ed.), *Essential Papers on Dreams* (pp. 452–473). New York: New York University Press.

Hobson, R. (1986). The autistic child's appraisal of expressions of emotion. *Journal of Child Psychology, Psychiatry and Related Disciplines, 27,* 321–342.

Hobson, R. (1990). On acquiring knowledge about people and the capacity to pretend: Response to Leslie (1987). *Psychological Review, 97,* 114–121.

Hochschild, A. (1979). Emotion work, feeling rules, and social structure. *American Journal of Sociology, 85,* 551–575.

Hubel, D. (1959). Single unit activity in striate cortex of unrestrained cats. *Journal of Physiology, 147,* 226–238.

Hubel, D., and Wiesel, T. (1959). Receptive fields of single neurones in the cat's striate cortex. *Journal of Physiology, 148,* 574–591.

Humphrey, N. (1984). *Consciousness regained: Chapters in the development of mind.* New York: Oxford University Press.

Izard, C., and Haynes, M. (1988). On the form and universality of the contempt expression: A challenge to Ekman and Friesen's claim to discovery. *Motivation and Emotion, 12,* 1–16.

Jackendoff, R. (1987). *Consciousness and the computational mind*. Cambridge,MA: MIT Press.

James, W. (1890). *The principles of psychology*. New York: Henry Holt.

Joseph, A. (1985). Bitemporal atrophy in a patient with Frégoli syndrome, syndrome of intermetamorphosis, and reduplicative paramnesia. *American Journal of Psychiatry, 142,* 146–147.

Jürgens, U., and Ploog, D. (1970). Cerebral representation of vocalization in the squirrel monkey. *Experimental Brain Re*search, *10,* 532–554.

Kaada, B., (1951). Somato-motor, autonomic and electrocorticographic responses to electrical stimulation of "rhinencephalic" and other structures in primates, cat and dog. *Acta Physiologica Scandinavica, 24* [Suppl. 83], 1–285.

Kanner, L. (1943). Autistic disturbances of affective contact, *Nervous Child, 2,* 217–250.

Kanner, L . (1944). Early infantile autism. *Journal of Pediatrics, 25,* 211–217.

Karakashian, S., Gyger, M., and Marler, P. (1988). Audience effects on alarm calling in chickens (*Gallus gallus*). *Journal of Comparative Psych*ology, *102,* 129–135.

Karmiloff-Smith, A., Klima, E., Bellugi, U., Grant, J., and Baron-Cohen, S. (1995). Is there a social module? Language, face processing, and theory of mind in individuals with Williams Syndrome. *Journal of Cognitive Neuroscience, 7,* 196–208.

Keller, H. (1954). *The story of my life*. Garden City, NY: Doubleday.

Kemper, T. (1987). How many emotions are there? Wedding the social and the autonomic components. *American Journal of Sociology, 93,* 263–289.

Kendrick, K., and Baldwin, B. (1987). Cells in temporal cortex of conscious sheep can respond preferentially to the sight of faces. *Science 236,* 448–450.

Kerckhoff, A., and Back, K. (1968). *The June bug*. New York: Appleton Century Crofts.

Kirkpatrick, J. (1985). Some Marquesan understandings of action and identity. In G.M. White, J. Kirkpatrick (Eds)., *Person, Self, and Experience: Exploring Pacific Ethnopsychologies* (pp. 80–120). Berkeley, CA: University of California Press.

Kling, A.S., and Brothers, L. (1992). The amygdala and social behavior. In J. Aggleton (Ed.), *The Amygdala: Neurobiological Aspects of Emotion, Memory, and Mental Dysfunction* (pp. 353–377). New York: Wiley-Liss.

Kling, A.S., Dicks, D., and Gurowitz, E. (1969). Amygdalectomy and social behavior in a caged-group of vervets (*C. aethiops*). In C.R. Carpenter and H.O. Hofer (Eds.), *Proceedings of the Second International Congress of Primatology, Vol. 1* (pp. 232–241). New York: Karger, Basel.

Kling, A.S., Lancaster, J., and Benitone, J. (1970). Amygdalectomy in the freeranging vervet (*Cercopithecus aethiops*). *Journal of Psychiatric Research, 7,* 191–199.

Kling, A.S., Lloyd, R., Tachiki, K., Prince, H., Klimenko, V., and Korneva, E. (1992). Effects of social separation on immune function and brain neuro-transmitters in Cebus monkey (*Cebus apella*). *Annals of the New York Academy of Science, 650,* 257–261.

Kling, A.S., and Steklis, H.D. (1976). A neural substrate for affiliative behavior in nonhuman primates. *Brain, Behavior and Evolution, 13,* 216–238.

Klüver, H., and Bucy, P.C. (1937). "Psychic blindness" and other symptoms following bilateral temporal lobectomy in rhesus monkeys. *American Journal of Physiology, 119,* 352–353.

Klüver, H., and Bucy, P.C. (1939). Preliminary analysis of functions of the temporal lobes in monkeys. *Archives of Neurology and Psychiatry, 42,* 979–1000.

Kolb, F. and Braun, J. (1995). Blindsight in normal observers. *Nature, 377,* 336–338.

Kraut, R., and Johnston, R. (1979). Social and emotional messages of smiling: An ethological approach. *Journal of Personality and Social Psychology, 37,* 1539–1553.

Kruesi, M., Rapoport, J., Hamburger, S., Hibbs, E., Potter, W., Lenane, M., and Brown, G. (1990). Cerebrospinal fluid monoamine metabolites, aggression, and impulsivity in disruptive behavior disorders of children and adolescents. *Archives of General Psychiatry, 47,* 419–426.

Kummer, H., Dasser, V., and Hoyningen-Huene, P. (1990). Exploring primate social cognition: Some critical remarks. *Behaviour,* 112(1–2): 84–98.

Langdell, T. (1978). Recognition of faces: An approach to the study of autism. *Journal of Child Psychology, Psychiatry, and Related Disciplines, 19,* 255–268.

Le Bon, G. (1903). *The Crowd* (p. 29). London, Fisher Unwin.

LeDoux, J. (1991). Emotion and the limbic system concept. *Concepts in Neuroscience (World Scientific), 2,* 169–199.

LeDoux, J. (1995.) In search of an emotional system in the brain: Leaping from fear to emotion and consciousness. In M. Gazzaniga (Ed.), *The Cognitive Neurosciences* (pp. 1049–1061). Cambridge: MIT Press.

Leekam, S., and Perner, J. (1991). Does the autistic child have a metarepresentational deficit? *Cognition, 40,* 203–218.

Leiter, K. (1974). Adhocing in the schools: A study of placement practices in the kindergartens of two schools. In A. Cicourel, K. Jennings, S. Jennings, K. Leiter, R. MacKay, H. Mehan, D. Roth (Eds.), *Language Use and School Performance* (pp. 17–75). New York: Academic Press.

Leiter, K. (1976). Teachers' use of background knowledge to interpret test scores. *Sociology of Education Journal, 49,* 59–65.

Leiter, K. (1980). *A primer on ethnomethodology.* New York: Oxford University Press.

Leonard, C.M., Rolls, E.T., Wilson, F.A.W., and Baylis, G.C. (1985). Neurons in the amygdala of the monkey with responses selective for faces. *Behavioral Brain Research, 15,* 159–176.

Linnoila, M., Virkkunen, M., Scheinin, M., Nuutila, A., Rimon, R., and Goodwin, F. (1983). Low cerebrospinal fluid 5-hydroxyindoleacetic acid concentration differentiates impulsive from nonimpulsive violent behavior. *Life Sciences, 33,* 2609–2614.

Locke, J. (1993). *The child's path to spoken language.* Cambridge, MA: Harvard University Press.

Macchi, G. (1989). Anatomical substrate of emotional reactions. In F. Boller, J. Grafman (Eds.), *Handbook of neuropsychology, v. 3.* (pp. 283–303). New York: Elsevier Scientific Publishers.

MacLean, P. (1952). Some psychiatric implications of physiological studies on the frontotemporal portion of the limbic system (visceral brain). *Electroencephalography and Clinical Neurophysiology, 4,* 407–418.

Malcolm, N. (1986). *Wittgenstein: Nothing is hidden.* Oxford: Basil Blackwell.

Malliaras, D., Kossovitsa, Y., and Christodoulou, G. (1978). Organic contributors to the intermetamorphosis syndrome. *American Journal of Psychiatry, 135,* 985–987.

McCarthy, E.D. (1989). Emotions are social things: An essay in the sociology of emotions. In D. Franks, E. McCarthy (Eds.), *The sociology of emotions: Original essays and research papers* (pp. 51–72). Greenwich, CT: JAI Press, Inc.

Mead, G.H. (1934). *Mind, self and society from the standpoint of a social behaviorist.* Chicago: The University of Chicago Press.

Mehlman, P., Higley, J., Faucher, I., Lilly, A., Taub, D., Vickers, J., Suomi, S., and Linnoila, M. (1995). Correlation of CSF 5–HIAA concentration with sociality and the timing of emigration in free-ranging primates. *American Journal of Psychiatry, 152,* 907–913.

Meltzoff, A. (1990). Foundations for developing a concept of self: The role of imitation in relating self to other and the value of social mirroring, social modeling, and self practice in infancy. In D. Cicchetti, M. Beeghly (Eds.), *The self in transition: Infancy to childhood* (pp. 139–164). Chicago: The University of Chicago Press.

Meltzoff, A., and Gopnik, A. (1993). The role of imitation in understanding persons and developing a theory of mind. In S. Baron-Cohen, H. Tager-Flusberg, D. Cohen (Eds.), *Understanding other minds: Perspectives from autism* (pp. 335–366). Oxford: Oxford University Press.

Meltzoff, A., Moore, M. (1977). Imitation of facial and manual gestures by human neonates. *Science, 198,* 75–78.

Miller, D. (1973). *George Herbert Mead: Self, language, and the world.* Austin, TX: University of Texas Press.

Morris, J., Frith, C., Perret, D., Rowland, D., Young, A., Calder, and Dolan, R. (1996). A differential neural response in the human amygdala to fearful and happy facial expressions. *Nature, 383,* 812–815.

Nahm, F. (1994). *Neuroethological investigation of the monkey amygdaloid complex.* Unpublished doctoral dissertation, University of California, San Diego.

Nahm, F., Albright, T., and Amaral, D. (1991). Neuronal responses of the monkey amygdaloid complex to dynamic visual stimuli. *Society for Neuroscience Abstracts, 17,* 473.

Nakamura, K., Mikami, A., and Kubota, K. (1992). Activity of single neurons in the monkey amygdala during performance of a visual discrimination task. *Journal of Neurophysiology, 67,* 1447–1463.

Nelson, K., and Seidman, S. (1984). Playing with scripts. In I. Bretherton (Ed.), *Symbolic play: The development of social understanding* (pp. 45–71). Orlando, FL: Academic Press.

Neville, H. (1990). Intermodal competition and compensation in development. Evidence from studies of the visual system in congenitally deaf adults. *Annals of the New York Academy of Science, 608,* 71–87.

Ojemann, G. (1990). Organization of language cortex derived from investigations during neurosurgery. *Seminars in Neuroscience, 2,* 297–305.

Oram, M., and Perrett, D.I. (1994). Responses of anterior superior temporal polysensory (STPa) neurons to "biological motion" stimuli. *Journal of Cognitive Neuroscience, 6,* 99–116.

Ortony, A., and Turner, T. (1990). What's basic about basic emotions? *Psychological Review, 97,* 315–331.

Panksepp, J. (1982). Toward a general psychobiological theory of emotions. *Behavioral and Brain Sciences, 5,* 407–467.

Papez, J. (1937). A proposed mechanism of emotion. *Archives of Neurology and Psychiatry, 38,* 725–743.

Passingham, R. (1975). Changes in size and organization of the brain in man and his ancestors, *Brain Behavior and Evolution, 11,* 73–90.

Patry, R., and Nespoulous, J. L. (1990). Discourse analysis in linguistics: Historical and theoretical background. In Y. Joanette, H. Brownell (Eds.), *Discourse ability and brain damage: Theoretical and empirical perspectives* (pp. 3–27). New York: Springer-Verlag.

Patterson, K., and Baddeley, A. (1977). When face recognition fails. *Journal of Experimental Psychology, 3,* 406–417.

Pawlby, S. (1977). Imitative interaction. In H. Schaffer (Ed.), *Studies in mother–infant interaction* (pp. 203–224). New York: Academic Press.

Penfield, W., and Rasmussen, T. (1950). *The cerebral cortex of man: A clinical study of localization of function.* New York: Macmillan.

Penfield, W., and Roberts, L. (1959). *Speech and brain mechanisms.* Princeton, NJ: Princeton University Press.

Perinbanayagam, R. (1990). How to do self with things. In S. Riggins (Ed.), *Beyond Goffman: Studies on communication, institution, and social interaction* (pp. 315–340). New York: Mouton de Gruyter.

Perinbanayagam, R. (1991). *Discursive acts.* New York: Aldine de Gruyter.

Perrett, D.I., Harries, M.H., Benson, P.J., Chitty, A.J., and Mistlin, A.J. (1990). Retrieval of structure from rigid and biological motion: An analysis of the visual responses of neurones in the macaque temporal cortex. In A.

Blake, T. Troscianko (Eds.), *AI and the Eye* (pp. 181–201). Chichester: John Wiley and Sons.

Perrett, D.I., Harries, M.H., Chitty, A.J., and Mistlin, A.J. (1990). Three stages in the classification of body movements by visual neurones. In H. B. Barlow, C. Blakemore, and M. Weston-Smith (Eds.), *Images and understanding* (pp. 94–107). London: Cambridge University Press.

Perrett, D.I., Heitanen, J., Oram, M., and Benson, P. (1992). Organization and function of cells responsive to faces in the temporal cortex. *Philosophical Transactions of the Royal Society of London Series B, 335,* 23–30.

Perrett, D.I., and Mistlin, A.J. (1990). Perception of facial characteristics by monkeys. In W. Stebbins, M.A. Berkley (Eds.), *Comparative perception, 2* (pp. 187–215). New York: Wiley and Sons.

Perrett, D.I., Rolls, E.T., and Caan, W. (1979). Temporal lobe cells of the monkey with visual responses selective for faces. *Neuroscience Letters [suppl. 3],* 358.

Perrett, D.I., Rolls, E.T., and Caan, W. (1982). Visual neurons responsive to faces in the monkey temporal cortex. *Experimental Brain Research, 47,* 329–342.

Perrett, D.I., Smith, P.A.J., Potter, D.D., Mistlin, A.J., Head, A.S., Milner, A.D. and Jeeves, M.A. (1984). Neurones responsive to faces in the temporal cortex: studies of functional organization, sensitivity to identity, and relation to perception. *Human Neurobiology, 3,* 197–208.

Perrett, D.I., Smith, P.A.J., Potter, D.D., Mistlin, A.J., Head, A.S., Milner, A.D., and Jeeves, M.A.(1985). Visual cells in the temporal cortex sensitive to face view and gaze direction. *Proceedings of the Royal Society of London Series B, 223,* 293–317.

Pigarev, I., Rizzolatti, G., and Scandolara, C. (1979). Neurons responding to visual stimuli in the frontal lobe of macaque monkeys. *Neuroscience Letters, 12,* 207–212.

Piven, J., Berthier, M., Starkstein, S., Nehme, E., Pearlson, G., and Folstein, S. (1990). Magnetic resonance imaging evidence for a defect of cerebral cortical development in autism. *American Journal of Psychiatry, 147,* 734–739.

Povinelli, D. and Eddy, T. (1996). What young chimpanzees know about seeing. *Monographs of the Society for Research in Child Development, 61,* 1–152.

Premack, D. (1988). "Does the chimpanzee have a theory of mind?" revisited. In R. Byrne, A. Whiten (Eds.), *Machiavellian intelligence: Social expertise and the evolution of intellect in monkeys, apes, and humans* (pp. 160–179). Oxford: Clarendon Press.

Premack, D., and Woodruff, G. (1978). Does the chimpanzee have a theory of mind? *Behavioral and Brain Sciences, 1,* 515–26.

Preuss, T. (1994). The argument from animals to humans in cognitive neuroscience. In M. Gazzaniga (Ed.), *The Cognitive neurosciences* (pp. 1227–1241). Cambridge: MIT Press.

Price, J., and Amaral, D. (1981). An autoradiographic study of the projections of the central nucleus of the monkey amygdala. *Journal of Neuroscience 1,* 1242–1259.

Provine, R. (1993). Laughter punctuates speech: Linguistic, social and gender contexts of laughter. *Ethology, 95,* 291–298.

Quine, W.V. (1969). *Ontological relativity and other essays.* New York: Columbia University Press.

Raleigh, M.J. (1976). *Brain and behavior: The effects of orbitofrontal lesions on behavior in vervet monkeys,* Unpublished doctoral dissertation. University of California, Berkeley.

Raleigh, M.J., and Brammer, G.L. (1993). Individual differences in serotonin–2 receptors and social behavior in monkeys. *Society for Neuroscience Abstracts, 19,* 592.

Raleigh, M.J., Brammer, G., Ritvo, E., Yuwiler, A., McGuire, M., and Geller, E. (1986). Effects of chronic fenfluramine on blood serotonin, cerebrospinal fluid metabolites, and behavior in monkeys. *Psychopharmacology, 90,* 503–508.

Raleigh, M.J., Brammer, G., Yuwiler, A., Flannery, J., McGuire, M., and Geller, E. (1980). Serotonergic influences on the social behavior of vervet monkeys (*Cercopithecus aethiops sabaeus*). *Experimental Neurology, 68,* 322–334.

Raleigh, M.J., McGuire, M., Brammer, G., Pollack, D., and Yuwiler, A. (1991). Serotonergic mechanisms promote dominance acquisition in adult male vervet monkeys. *Brain Research, 559,* 181–190.

Raleigh, M.J., and Steklis, H.D. (1981). Effects of orbital frontal and temporal neocortical lesions on affiliative behavior of vervet monkeys. *Experimental Neurology, 73,* 378–389.

Ramachandran, V. (1990). Interactions between motion, depth, color and form: The utilitarian theory of perception. In C. Blakemore (Ed.), *Vision: Coding and efficiency* (pp. 346–360). Cambridge: Cambridge University Press.

Recanzone, G., Schreiner, C., and Merzenich, M. (1993). Plasticity in the frequency representation of primary auditory cortex following discrimination training in adult owl monkeys. *Journal of Neuroscience, 13,* 87–103.

Révész, G. (1956). *The origins and prehistory of language.* New York: Philosophical Library.

Rinn, W. (1984). The neuropsychology of facial expression: A review of the neurological and psychological mechanisms for producing facial expressions. *Psychological Bulletin, 95,* 52–77.

Rizzolatti, G., Fadiga, L., Gallese, V. and Fogassi, L. (1996). Premotor cortex and the recognition of motor actions. *Cognitive Brain Research, 3,* 131–141.

Robinson, B. (1967). Vocalization evoked from forebrain in *Macaca mulatta. Physiology and Behavior, 2,* 345–354.

Robinson, B., and Mishkin, M. (1968). Penile erection evoked from forebrain structures in *Macaca mulatta. Archives of Neurology, 19,* 184–198.

Rolls, E.T. (1981). Responses of amygdaloid neurons in the primate. In Y. Ben-Ari (Ed.), *The amygdaloid complex* (pp. 383–393). Amsterdam: Elsevier.

Rolls, E.T. (1995). Learning mechanisms in the temporal lobe visual cortex. *Behavioural Brain Research, 66,* 177–185.

Rorty, R. (1979). *Philosophy and the mirror of nature.* Princeton, NJ: Princeton University Press.

Ross, E. (1981). The aprosodias: Functional-anatomic organization of the affective components of language in the right hemisphere. *Archives of Neurology, 38,* 561–569.

Ross, E., and Mesulam, M-M. (1979). Dominant language functions of the right hemisphere? Prosody and emotional gesturing. *Archives of Neurology, 36,* 144–148.

Sacks, H. (1984). On doing "being ordinary." In M. Atkinson, J. Heritage (Eds.), *Structures of social action: Studies in conversation analysis,* (pp. 413–429). Cambridge: Cambridge University Press.

Sacks, H., Schegloff, E., and Jefferson, G. (1974). A simplest systematics for the organization of turn-taking for conversation. *Language, 50,* 696–735.

Salmelin, R., Hari, R., Lounasmaa, O., and Sams, M. (1994). Dynamics of brain activation during picture naming. *Nature, 368,* 463–465.

Sanghera, M.F., Rolls, E.T., and Roper-Hall, A. (1979). Visual response of neurons in the dorsolateral amygdala of the alert monkey. *Experimental Neurology, 63,* 61–62.

Saver, J.L., and Damasio, A. (1991). Preserved access and processing of social knowledge in a patient with acquired sociopathy due to ventromedial frontal damage. *Neuropsychologia, 29,* 1241–9.

Scaife, M., and Bruner, J. (1975). The capacity for joint visual attention in the infant. *Nature, 253,* 265–266.

Schafer, R. (1992). *Retelling a life: Narration and dialogue in psychoanalysis.* New York: Basic Books.

Schank, R. (1990). *Tell me a story: A new look at real and artificial memory.* New York: Charles Scribner's Sons.

Schreiner, L., and Kling, A. (1953). Behavioral changes following rhinencephalic injury in cat. *Journal of Neurophysiology, 16,* 643–659.

Schreiner, L., and Kling, A. (1956). Rhinencephalon and behavior. *American Journal of Physiology, 184,* 468–490.

Schutz, A. (1962). In M. Natanson (Ed.), *The problem of social reality, Collected papers* (vol. 1). The Hague: Martinus Nijhoff.

Schwaber, E. (1990). Interpretation and the therapeutic action of psychoanalysis. *International Journal of Psychoanalysis, 71,* 229–240.

Shapin, S. (1994). *A social history of truth: Civility and science in seventeenth-century England.* Chicago: University of Chicago Press.

Shapin, S., and Schaffer, S. (1985). *Leviathan and the air-pump: Hobbes, Boyle, and the experimental life.* Princeton, NJ: Princeton University Press.

Sigman, M., Kasari, C., Kwon, J., and Yirmiya, N. (1992). Responses to the negative emotions of others by autistic, mentally retarded and normal children. *Child Development, 63,* 769–807.

Signer, S. (1987). Capgras' syndrome: The delusion of substitution. *Journal of Clinical Psychiatry, 48,* 147–150.

Sillito, A., Jones, H., Gerstein, G., and West, D. (1994). Feature-linked synchronization of thalamic relay cell firing induced by feedback from the visual cortex. *Nature, 369,* 479–482.

Silva, J., and Leong, G. (1991). A case of "subjective" Frégoli syndrome. *Journal of Psychiatry and Neuroscience, 16,* 103–105.

Silva, J., Leong, G., and Shaner, A. (1990). A classification system for misidentification syndromes. *Psychopathology, 23,* 27–32.

Silva, J., Leong, G., and Shaner, A. (1991). The syndrome of intermetamorphosis. *Psychopathology, 24,* 158–165.

Silva, J., Leong, G., and Weinstock, R. (1991). Misidentification syndrome and male pseudocyesis. *Psychosomatics, 32,* 228–230.

Singer, M. (1980). Signs of the self: An exploration in semiotic anthropology. *American Anthropologist, 82,* 485–507.

Spence, D. (1982). *Narrative truth and historical truth: Meaning and interpretation in psychoanalysis.* New York: W.W. Norton.

Stent, G. (1975). Limits to the scientific understanding of man. *Science, 187,* 1052–1057.

Stephan, H., and Andy, O. (1970). The allocortex in primates. In C. Noback, W. Montagna (Eds.), *The Primate Brain* (pp. 109–135). New York: Appleton-Century-Crofts.

Stephan, H., Frahm, H., and Baron, G. (1987). Comparison of brain structure volumes in insectivora and primates VII. Amygdaloid components. *Journal für Hirnforschung, 28,* 571–584.

Stern, D. (1985). *The Interpersonal world of the infant: A view from psychoanalysis and developmental psychology.* New York: Basic Books.

Stolorow, R., and Atwood, G. (1992). *Contexts of being: The intersubjective foundations of psychological life.* Hillsdale, NJ: Analytic Press.

Strawson, P., (1959). Persons. In *Individuals: An essay in descriptive metaphysics* (pp. 87–116). London: Methuen and Co.

Sullivan, H.S. (1953). *The interpersonal theory of psychiatry.* New York: W.W. Norton.

Sullivan, K., and Winner, E. (1993). Three-year-olds' understanding of mental states: The influence of trickery. *Journal of Experimental Child Psychology, 56,* 135–48.

Tager-Flusberg, H. (1992). Autistic children's talk about psychological states: Deficits in the early acquisition of a theory of mind. *Child Development, 63,* 161–172.

Tager-Flusberg, H. (1993). What language reveals about the understanding of minds in children with autism. In S. Baron-Cohen, H. Tager-Flusberg, D. Cohen (Eds.), *Understanding Other Minds: Perspectives from Autism* (pp. 138–157). Oxford: Oxford University Press.

Tager-Flusberg, H., Calkins, S., Nolin, T., Baumberger, T., Anderson, M., and Chadwick-Dias, A. (1990). A longitudinal study of language acquisition in autistic and Down syndrome children. *Journal of Autism and Developmental Disorders, 20,* 1–21.

Tooby, J., and DeVore, I. (1987). The reconstruction of hominid behavioral evolution through strategic modeling. In W. G. Kinzey (Ed.), *The evolution of human behavior: Primate models.* Albany: SUNY Press.

Tranel, D., and Hyman, B. (1990). Neuropsychological correlates of bilateral amygdala damage. *Archives of Neurology, 47,* 349–355.

Treffert, D. (1989). *Extraordinary people: Understanding "idiot savants."* New York: Harper and Row.

Trevarthen, C. (1979). The tasks of consciousness: How could the brain do them? In *Brain and Mind (Ciba Foundation Symposium 69),* (pp. 187–215). Amsterdam: Excerpta Medica.

Trevarthen, C., and Logotheti, K. (1989). Child and culture: Genesis of co-operative knowing. In A. Gellatly, D. Rogers, J. Sloboda (Eds.), *Cognition and social worlds* (pp. 37–56). Oxford: Clarendon Press.

Ursin, H. (1972). Limbic control of emotional behavior. In E. Hitchcock, L. Laitinen, K. Vaernet (Eds.), *Psychosurgery* (pp. 34–45). Springfield, Illinois: Charles C. Thomas.

Uzgiris, I., Benson, J., Kruper, J., and Vasek, M. (1989). Establishing action-environment correspondences: Contextual influences on imitative interactions between mothers and infants. In J. Lockman, N. Hazen (Eds.), *Action in Social Context* (pp. 103–127). New York: Plenum.

Van Hoesen, G. (1982, October). The parahippocampal gyrus: New observations regarding its cortical connections in the monkey. *Trends in Neuroscience, 5,* 345–350.

Van Hoesen, G., and Pandya, D. (1975). Some connections of the entorhinal (area 28) and perirhinal (area 35) cortices of the rhesus monkey. I. Temporal lobe afferents. *Brain Research, 95,* 1–24.

Van Hoesen, G., Pandya, D., and Butters, N. (1972). Cortical afferents to the entorhinal cortex of the rhesus monkey. *Science, 175,* 1471–1473.

Van Hoesen, G., Pandya, D., and Butters, N. (1975). Some connections of the entorhinal (area 28) and perirhinal (area 35) cortices of the rhesus monkey. II. Frontal lobe afferents. *Brain Research, 95,* 25–38.

Weeks, S., and Hobson, R. (1987). The salience of facial expression for autistic children. *Journal of Child Psychology and Psychiatry and Allied Disciplines, 28,* 137–152.

Weinberger, N. (1993). Retuning the brain by fear conditioning. In M. Gazzaniga (Ed.), *The cognitive neurosciences* (pp. 1071–1089). Cambridge, MA: MIT Press.

Weiskrantz, L. (1956). Behavioral changes associated with ablation of the amygdaloid complex in monkeys. *Journal of Comparitive Physiology and Psychology, 49,* 381–391.

Wertsch, J. (1985). *Vygotsky and the social formation of mind.* Cambridge, MA: Harvard University Press.

Whiten, A., and Byrne, R. (1989). Machiavellian monkeys: Cognitive evolution and the social world of primates. In A. Gellatly, D. Rogers, J. Sloboda (Eds.), *Cognition and Social Worlds* (pp. 22–36). Oxford: Clarendon Press.

Wieder, D. (1974). *Language and social reality: The case of telling the convict code.* The Hague: Mouton.

Wilson, F., Ó Scalaidhe, S., and Goldman-Rakic, P. (1993). Dissociation of object and spatial processing domains in primate prefrontal cortex, *Science* 260: 1955–1958.

Wimmer, H., and Perner, J. (1983). Belief about beliefs: Representation and constraining function of wrong beliefs in young children's understanding of deception. *Cognition, 13,* 103–128.

Wimmer, H., and Weichbold, V. (1994). Children's theory of mind: Fodor's heuristics examined. *Cognition, 53,* 45–57.

Wing, L. (1988a). Preface: The autistic continuum. In L. Wing (Ed.), *Aspects of Autism: Biological Research* (pp. v–viii). Oxford, UK: Alden Press.

Wing, L. (1988b). Autism: possible clues to the underlying pathology—1. Clinical facts. In L. Wing (Ed.), *Aspects of Autism: Biological Research* (pp. 1–10). Oxford, UK: Alden Press.

Wittgenstein, L. (1953). *Philosophical investigations.* (G.E.M. Anscombe, Trans.). Oxford: Blackwell.

Wittling, W., and Roschmann, R. (1993). Emotion-related hemisphere asymmetry: Subjective emotional responses to laterally presented films. *Cortex, 29,* 431–448.

Yamane, S., Kaji, S., and Kawano, K. (1988). What facial features activate face neurons in the inferotemporal cortex of the monkey? *Experimental Brain Research, 73,* 209–214.

Yirmiya, N., Sigman, M., Kasari, C., and Mundy, P. (1992). Empathy and cognition in high-functioning children with autism. *Child Development, 63,* 150–160.

Young, A. (1992). Face recognition impairments. *Philosophical Transactions of the Royal Society of London Series B, 335,* 47–54.

Young, A., Aggleton, J., Hellawell, D., Johnson, M., Broks, P., and Hanley, J. (1995). Face processing impairments after amygdalotomy. *Brain, 118,* 15–24.

Young, M., and Yamane, S. (1992). Sparse population coding of faces in the inferotemporal cortex. *Science, 256,* 1327–1331.

Zaitchik, D. (1990). When representations conflict with reality: The preschooler's problem with false beliefs and "false" photographs. *Cognition, 35,* 41–68.

Index